My Other Car Is An Ambulance

Scott Eberhart

My Other Car Is An Ambulance

Editor: Esther Baruch

First published: December 18, 2023

Copyright © 2023 Scott Eberhart

ISBN: 979-8-218-32183-3

To my wife and children:

Without you I would not have believed I could.

To the patients in my head:

Apparently, you aren't leaving.

CONTENTS

Preface

These stories are the highlights of over thirty years of calls. I have met, treated, watched die, helped live, and made a difference in the lives of thousands more people. This is what it's like being a paramedic... over the long term.

The point of this book depends on who you are as a reader. If you're looking to enter the business, this is what you're getting into. If you already live the life, you'll recognize yourself and your patients on these pages. If you are a member of the general reading public who only sees pre-hospital emergency medicine on TV and as the ambulance rushes by, this is a look inside.

The chapters may seem rapid-fire and disjointed. That is my intention. It's what the job is like. As a paramedic, I thrive in the chaotic and fragmented moments of someone else's worst day. I meet a patient and their family for, at most, twenty minutes to an hour. Usually I don't know what happens after I leave. I don't seek the outcome of the illness or injury I strived to improve. I'll give you all I've got while I'm with you. But once the ambulance is cleaned up, I'm off to the next call and they get all I have.

So, strap in. Enjoy the ride. It gets bumpy.

CHAPTER 1

It's Strange....

Last night I stood outside a man's bedroom where he lay alone, face down, sprawled atop the clutter, mid-frantic attempt at . . . something. Stepping inside, I only needed the heart monitor.

I balanced my left boot on a pillow, then found an open bit of carpet for my right boot. It was a bit of a stretch, but the clutter was such there were no other options near enough to the body. The heart monitor shared the space on the pillow, resting against my leg, tilted up, so I could see the screen.

Placing the stickers on his back, I ran the strip. The cops and medics and firefighters all stood outside the room, tense, just in case we were all wrong.

The bullet hole, about the size of a pencil, pierced the back of his shaved head.

And that was it.

No dramatic music, no perfect camera angle juxtaposing this tragedy against the softer sides of his life. Most strange, as I took back the wires, stepped gingerly out of the room, and walked downstairs past the neighbors, most strange was there was no cut to a commercial.

CHAPTER 2

Surf Rescue

1704 hours.

"Unit dispatch. Engine 23, Engine 34 on SR34, Engine 18 on SR18, Truck 14, Truck 18, Rescue Squad 1, Medic 76, RC2, and Battalion 7 respond, with the Coast Guard, to Ocean Beach, Stairwell 15 for the Surf Rescue. Respond on A2, your tach channel is A7."

"Hey, Scott. Did you hear that?"

Mike's question drew my attention away from the mushrooms I was slicing for dinner.

"No. What was it?"

"They've got a surf rescue."

"I wonder if they'll want the rescue watercraft. Should we let Jerry know?"

"Sure, I'll give a holler upstairs."

Mike walked to the other room for the P.A.

"Hey, Lieutenant. A surf rescue is going down off Ocean Beach. They haven't called us yet. Just letting you know."

Mike came back to the kitchen and picked up a knife to attack the carrots.

Jerry sauntered into the communication room, over to the computer, and brought up the dispatch screen.

The phone rang and Jerry picked up the receiver.

"Station 16, Lieutenant Keohane."

He listened for a few seconds.

"Yeah. Okay. We'll get 'em going."

He put the phone down, reached for the P.A. system, and pushed the button.

"Okay, guys. Everybody. Let's go. They want the skis and boat for a surf rescue. Kids into the surf at Ocean Beach. Saddle up."

Mike and I left the knives and ran to the rigs. He on the truck, me on the engine.

The assigned swimmers for the day, Dennis, John, and Sasha, shed clothes as they ran toward the rigs. They tried to change into their wetsuits before we hit the road.

"Hey, Sasha," I said. "Do you want me to jump the driver's seat for you so you can change on the way over?"

"Yeah. Thanks." She said with her distinct Aussie drawl. "Just keep your eyes on the road."

She dropped her pants to stand in shorts. Sasha, like anybody else in the house, never passed up a chance to poke a jab for fun.

"Aw, come on. Do you think I want to watch Dennis strip off? Throw me a bone."

"Shut up and drive."

"Yes, ma'am."

I opened the door of the fire engine, grabbed the steering wheel, and pulled myself into the driver's seat.

With everyone on board, I turned on the lights, tapped the horn a few times, warning people who might be out of sight on the sidewalk, and started into the street.

We beat the truck out the door. But that's as it should be. The engine should always beat the truck.

Tearing through the streets, I blasted the air horn with my left heel while Jerry controlled the siren from his seat. Sasha and Dennis did their best to pull on the tight wet suits and not fall over.

Once at the marina, Jerry handed me the keys and I ran down the dock to prep the skis with Mike's help. We pulled the tarps and ran the cables out of the locks. Sasha and Dennis, helmets on, life jackets tight, their swim fins strapped to waist belts, climbed on the watercraft and fired them up. John scrambled on behind Sasha while Mike and I moved to the front of the skis and pushed them off into the waters of the marina.

The two skis, and three firefighters aboard them, motored off toward the bay, rescue sleds trailing tightly behind. The Rescue Boat cleared its mooring and followed. Our job finished, the rest of us from the engine stood on the dock listening to Jerry's radio, hoping for nothing bad to happen in the ebb of a gorgeous May evening.

And that is what happened: The call stayed open. The Rescue boat combed deeper waters off Ocean Beach alongside the Coast Guard, while the watercraft weaved their way in and out around Seal Rocks, matching tidal flow.

Jerry, his turnout pants with the suspenders hanging loose to his knees, propped his left hand on his hip, his right dangling the radio down by his side; his familiar stance.

"Okay, folks. This thing is going to play out for a while. Get comfy. There's only two hours till sunset when they have to come in."

And finally, they did. Rounding the corner into the marina with a slow, exhausted motor, Sasha and Dennis had been driving for two hours, John straddling the seat behind Sasha. I stood ready with the hose to put fresh water through the skis and boat after hauling them onto their moorings.

Back at the house, we traded bits of information.

Greg, the driver of the truck, piped in.

"He just walked them into the water. Guy's fucking crazy. He drowned his own kids in the ocean."

Will, another truckie, asked, "Who called 911?"

Jerry offered that answer.

"Supposedly, some guy, at Ocean Beach with his son, saw the guy acting weird with his kids right at the surf line. He took off to call 911. The dad grabbed up the kids and walked right into the surf with them while the other guy went looking for a phone."

We were all shaken from the absurdity.

I stopped putting forks and knives around the table.

"How old were they? Anybody heard that?"

Greg's booming voice rose above the din of the TV and gathering of bodies in the kitchen.

"I'm hearing one was about two years old and the other about four."

"Four!" I said. "How can you make a four-year-old jump in the ocean without a fight? That doesn't make sense."

The swimmers came back downstairs after taking showers. Sasha, her blonde hair still hanging wet below her shoulders, put the finished salad on the table as we all sat down for dinner.

"We were out there for two hours. That water was damn cold and the spray kept hitting us in the face. I couldn't see a thing half the time. We need some glasses or something."

"I use safety glasses for starting IV's," I offered. "You should try them next time you go out. That might work."

"Yeah, that might work. Damn spray starts to hurt like needles after a while."

I continued, "What did they have you doing? It sounded like they were working you in around Seal Rocks and the Cliff House."

"Yeah, we were right up against the rocks. Trying to maneuver those skis in tight like that is tough. Then a wave would come up and throw us into the rocks. Scratched the hell out of one of the skis."

"But you didn't find a thing. The kids or the dad, I mean."

"No. We ran from Seal Rocks all the way in through the Gate. Nothing. They aren't there. They either dropped like a stone, or the tide's taken them who knows where."

"That sucks," I said.

Dinner was eaten with plenty of talk and speculation.

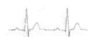

"Units dispatch. E16, M28, RC2, Battalion 4 to Hyde Street Pier for the Evaluation. Respond on A2, your tach channel is A14."

2206 hours.

I read the text on the engine's computer while we drove through the darkened streets. The Coast Guard had found one of the kids and brought him ashore at Hyde Street Pier.

I pulled on my gloves slowly. I knew why we'd been called. As the paramedic, I was the only one really necessary. And we wouldn't need an ambulance.

We pulled up and I stepped out of the rig. I grabbed the medical bag and the heart monitor. I grabbed the medical bag because I always grab the medical bag and I couldn't go down there having given up before even seeing the kid, but I wouldn't need it.

I walked past the news lights and cameras and down the pier with a firm pace. After passing a building I turned right and met a small gathering of people. Two, I noticed, wore the orange life vests of the Coast Guard crew. They appeared barely old enough to drive but they'd brought me my patient. I could only imagine what method they used to pull the kid out of the water.

I turned and looked down. Illuminated by the harsh light of a bare bulb and its metal shade, a child, about two years old, lay on a blue plastic tarp. His limbs, splayed wide, opened his body to the cold damp of the pier.

Oh, my God. He's naked.

The heart monitor hung from my left shoulder. The bulky medical bag hung on my right.

All day long, the horrific story of this boy unraveled on the news, showing the family picture the media had found. The oldest one held the younger one, almost toppling over as they laughed. They both giggled as the photo forever suspended them from falling to the floor.

I think I had the younger kid, judging by his height and compared to the picture in my mind. It was hard to tell. They both smiled and looked happy in their play clothes. Tonight, this one lay motionless, his head to the left and . . .

He's naked.

My brain called.

Scott, do something. You're the reason we're here.

I dropped to my knees and this brought me closer to the boy. His body had lengthened as he neared the end of his diaper days but he still had the chub of an infant in his cheeks. His eyes . . . oh, they were half-closed in a frozen stillness from the frigid water.

Again, my brain called.

Stop. This is simple. Declare this child dead.

Mentally, I ran through the County Protocols and accessed the policy, "Death In The Field." Contained within stated criteria such as decapitation, decomposition, and "separation from the body of either brain, liver, or heart." If that were the case, I could stop my exam and declare him dead. Not so here. He could possibly fill the requirement for rigor mortis but he'd been pulled from the water. He was cold and stiff from that alone.

My head swirled again. This wasn't working. Kneeling next to the boy, I was the closest person to him. However, I was still a spectator, someone who had been listening to the news all day about a father, recently divorced and, in his grief, feeling he needed to keep the children from the mother... forever. I was no better than any of us at the end of the pier. No, actually, I was worse. My job allowed me to sidle up next to the scintillating stuff our society loved to see. I was given that privilege because I was supposed to do something to make the problem better. Now? I was another gawker, up close and personal. This wouldn't do. He deserved more. I gave in and moved closer to the boy. Closer to my patient.

He was a child, a two-year-old child. His eyes were half-closed and he lay with a stillness my mind believed could be interrupted with a breath at any moment. I found myself waiting for that breath. His face was passive, some would say peaceful.

No, not peaceful. Peace is gained with knowledge of goodness and serenity. This child had that torn from him as he was carried, like overstuffed luggage, into the cold waters of the Pacific Ocean. He knew nothing of peace.

No, his face was simply — lifeless. The warmth and beauty of the two-year-old child who woke this morning was gone, far from this pier, away from the yellow glare of a simple bulb, definitely not lying sprawled and exposed on a blue tarp.

He's naked. He must have been so cold.

With a gloved hand I reached for the heart monitor, the cords and the patches attached. I peeled off a sticker and put the white-colored lead below his right shoulder. I felt the icy, rubbery skin through my glove. I followed with the black lead to his left shoulder.

A voice spoke up from behind me, one of the Coasties. "You know . . . he's been in the water over five hours."

The unspoken meaning: *What are you doing? He's dead.*

"Yes, I know. This one's going to court."

I put the red lead on his left side and flipped the switch on the monitor.

I pressed the record button and the paper fed out, a continuous, heartless, cold pace. The date and time were on the top of the strip and the paper held only one other marking: A simple, concluding, final, straight line.

2216 hours.

I stopped the tape. It was official. The boy was dead.

I wanted there to be more, there had to be more.

He's naked.

I wanted to hold him. I wanted the warmth from my body to spill over to his. This was wrong. He was only two.

I finally pulled the leads from his chest and wrapped the cords back into the pouch. Jerry stood over me.

He read the pain on my face, "What do you need?"

"A patient care form please."

I had to record the event for the medical examiner.

I sat on the pier next to my patient as I wrote. He was still mine. He belonged to me. I would let him go when I finished. My pen scratched out the story.

I wanted to write about his last birthday party. I wanted my pen to describe the giggles I'd added to the picture from the media. No. My story told of him being carried into fifty-five degree water; without any mercy, dying very soon; then floating for five hours before being scooped from the water and laid out for me to examine. It ended as my pen etched, "2216. Declared dead."

I finished as the medical examiner's crew arrived. I stood, tore off the copies and handed them the strip showing asystole. I looked down at my boy, one more time.

He now belonged to someone else.

Back at the firehouse I undressed for bed. In the bright lights of the bathroom I mechanically brushed and flossed. Finished, the next step was toward the darkened dormitory. Tonight, for me, the dorm also held the vision of a drowned boy. Instead, I sat on the bench, next to the lockers.

Dennis walked in.

I asked with a quiet voice, "What are you doing up? It's midnight."

"I can't sleep. That call is in my head."

"Yeah. I know what you mean."

Dennis sat on the bench next to me. We both leaned our elbows on our knees while he talked to the floor.

"The kid was lying on the tarp. He was lying there . . . with sand on his legs."

Dennis stopped. I searched back in my mind and tried to remember the sand clinging to the boy's legs. That memory hadn't stuck with me.

He spoke again, softly, "I was standing behind you as you worked on the kid. I was so angry." Now clipped and crisp. "I was so fucking angry."

We both fell silent, his anger poking at my own pain.

Dennis started, once again.

"I couldn't be a paramedic, man. I don't know how you do it. If the dad would have been there right then, I would have choked the living shit out of him. I'm glad they never found him. I mean, that kid seemed about as old as my two-year-old. Is that how old he was?

"Yeah. That's what I wrote down."

"Who would do that to a two-year-old kid?"

In my mind the child lay open on the tarp. Looking back, wrapping him up seemed better. Would have kept him warm. Yet, leaving him exposed felt necessary to allow an underscore, among us professionals, of the futility of covering a dead child. It also permitted us an angry, silent scream over what had been done to him.

"I don't understand it, either, Dennis. For me, pronouncing him dead is not what's getting to me."

I felt the impassiveness of that statement and reviewed the efficiency with which I performed tonight. I walked up, put patches on a kid's skin, pulled a strip, and wrote a chart. I questioned whether I had stopped caring: Call 'em dead and move on. But now, I sat in a lighted locker room because I couldn't go into the darkened dorm to face my patient.

"For me, I keep picturing those kids, both of them, at the beach with their dad."

Oh, God. That was it. I could feel it, the chord strumming the pain within me. I forced myself to strike it again.

"They were at the water with him, out for an evening walk by the sea. Just daddy and the kids."

I stopped as my mind took me to Ocean Beach.

"What did he say first? What could he say? 'Okay, children, we're going for a swim.'"

The pain rose in my throat as I saw two children, the confusion beginning in their eyes. They couldn't have heard Daddy right.

"Let's go. Into the water."

He grabbed the youngest one and stripped him of clothing, even the diaper, baring him naked on the sand in the chill of the evening.

The other stared, disbelieving, the confusion increasing along with a growing fear. His voice cried in confused whimpers, tears streamed down his face.

"Why Daddy? We don't want to go swimming."

The tears spilled over and rolled down my face.

"Do it! I'm your father, do as I say!"

They stripped off and stood on the sand at the water's

edge because you always do as Daddy asks.

"Daddy, I'm cold."

I cried out and released the pain as the horror washed over me.

"He used them! He used his children's trust against them. They stripped naked because Dad said so and he grabbed them up and walked into the water. How could he use his children's innocence and trust to kill them?"

I sobbed uncontrollably into my hands with Dennis at my side.

My tears slowed.

"I have to dry up. We could get a call and I can't go out there looking like I've been bawling my eyes out."

Dennis responded in a soothing voice.

"It's okay. You do what you need to do."

He was right. The pain burned as it rose but it was healing to let it go. My mind returned to the ocean, now my own children before me, their eyes filled with trust. Children believe in their parents. I cried into my hands, while sitting on the bench, in the locker room of the fire station.

The next day I showered and dressed to leave work. Normally, I went home and began my day with my wife and children. Today, I was drawn to Stairwell 15. I parked my car and walked to the media frenzy, stepping over the snakes of cable. I didn't know what I wanted from here. I needed to be close, to see in a different way, the beach entrance I had used so many times myself. I stood next to the Command Center trailer, out of the way, while the mayor was interviewed, the Chief of Department standing at his side.

After the cameras finished, the Chief glanced around and saw me. She knew I was on the call last night. She made her way to me, decked out in her Class A uniform, the gold of her rank prominently displayed.

Our eyes met.

"Are you okay?"
I couldn't hold back the tears as I answered.
"No. I'm not."

Later in the day I headed over to pick up the kids from school. They were so sweet and I could use their love.

On the way to the car I said, "Hey. Dad had a rough time at work yesterday. I could use a hug."

"Sure, Dad."

And I got a quick, confused, half-hearted hug from both of them before we reached the car parked at the curb and they began.

"Just get in and scoot over."

"No, you go around to the other side. I was here first."

"Why should I have to go around? Get in and scoot over. Dad! She won't let me . . . ."

Back to reality.

CHAPTER 3

Cleveland, Ohio

Paramedics are cool. They speed around town in ambulances decked out in lights and sirens. If you ask them, they've got the greatest stories. They're on the news, wheeling people away on gurneys and saving lives on the way to the hospital.

With such a great job, why is it impressive to find a paramedic who's still in after ten years? Why do the divorce and suicide rates for paramedics hover alongside cops? I started this job thirty years ago excited to show up every day. Now I wonder if I should step away before I kill someone and find out I don't care. In other words,

"Hello, my name is Scott and I am a paramedic."

Paramedicine is an addiction. The excitement, the drama, the life and death struggles draw the moth to the flame. Inside, next to the tragedies and thrills, the moth thinks it thrives best. The heat given off feels good, soothing in its warmth, feeding the addict.

Sometimes the moth dives in and is killed instantly by the burning center. Other times, most of the time, its wings are slowly singed. The moth may survive to exit with stories of a thrilling life, the scars seared in to prove the tales. Or the wings melt and deform, curl and misshape, until they can no longer support flight and the moth falls away, straining to touch the glory once so close, so wondrous and so . . . tasty.

Thirty-eight thousand times, give or take a few group stabbings and multiple car wrecks, I've saved my little corner of the world, although that's not completely accurate. I haven't even tried to save the world. Over the last thirty years I have walked in the door and said, "What can I do to make your problem better?"

That's what I love to do, what I'm good at. But, and it's a question coming up more frequently for me, while obviously avoiding the burning center, how do I recognize when my wings are becoming seared beyond the point needed to support flight? How do I distinguish the difference between another memorable moment, another intriguing tale, or another cut on an integral support to my sanity?

It didn't start out this way.

Spring Semester, 1981
Stow High School, Sophomore Year
Drafting Class
Instead of drawing a cylinder

"I hate sales, don't like business, working in an office would drive me nuts . . . ."

That was me figuring out what I *didn't* want to do for a career. I'd already run a big, fat zero on the list of things I *did* want to do.

Later that month, I took a CPR course for extra credit in biology and discovered I liked learning about the human body, how it worked, and how to keep a broken one going. Combined with life-or-death tension? Very cool.

Hey, that's a paramedic. I can do *that* for a living.

A little reading in the library and I found out becoming an Emergency Medical Technician would only take one semester at the junior college. Hold the EMT card for six months and I could sign up for a paramedic course.

A friend from high school, Chris, had gotten her EMT certification the year before and been hired by an ambulance company in Cleveland. She invited me to do a ride-along with her. This was the best! I could ask questions; put my hands on the actual equipment, and experience, for real, what being a paramedic was all about.

We arrived for her shift and she began her ambulance checkout by lifting the hood and checking the oil with me right at her side.

She pulled the dipstick but stopped at the end.

"You can go look inside. You don't have to wait for me."

Yippee!

I climbed inside the ambulance where her partner busily inventoried the open medical boxes on the end of the gurney. Around him, recessed lighting erased all hint of shadow; clear plastic and white dominated, suggesting an air of efficiency; and the tools of medicine lay pressed into every cranny. Boxes and needles lay retrievable with only an inch of movement. Cabinets, stuffed with mysterious unknowns, had only sliding plastic doors preventing contents from spilling onto the floor and the gurney.

My experience with medical stuff so far had been the doctor's office: Tongue depressors, cotton swabs, and shots for kindergarten. Here, I stepped into an alternate universe enclosed in a box on wheels.

I remember asking about everything. Why are you checking this? Why are you doing that? The medic, displaying incredible patience with my barrage of questions, allowed the cabinets to present their inventories. The bags and boxes, each one opened for inspection, burst with tools and medicines as he moved smoothly from item to item, adjusting, pushing, peering, and counting.

Then there was the driving.

This wasn't driving an automobile and they did not cover this in Driver's Ed. I distinctly remember sitting in a trailer behind the school, belted into a mock-up car with its steering wheel. On the screen in front of us played a video showing just the hood of a 1960s sedan topped with a garish hunk of metal crudely shaped into an eagle, like the figurehead for some grand, sea-going vessel. We sat in the darkened trailer "cruising" a neighborhood street while perilous soccer balls rolled from the blind spot between cars. Spinning our wheel only illuminated a light at the teacher's console but did nothing to alter our heading down the serene backwaters of suburban tranquility.

Now, in the back of the ambulance, perched on the seat, I held on as we careened around corners, made a mockery of the speed limit, drove straight into oncoming traffic and violated the entire Driver's Ed class rule book in the space of three city blocks. I realized the teacher had held back on us. There was more, so much more.

I craned my neck to gaze out the windshield as we blazed down a Cleveland street. The siren's continuous scream split the air: A distraction properly rated as unsportsmanlike. Cars moved to the side, sort of, and reflections of the lights flashed in the store windows we passed. Chris, in the passenger seat, called out "Clear right!" ensuring our safe travel through the red lights, at least from her side of the ambulance.

The paramedic was so cool. With one hand on the steering wheel, weaving between cars, he pulled a cigarette from the pack and flipped it to his lips. He leaned over and fished the lighter from his back pocket, avoided a truck, then lit up. His deplorable and dangerous driving, not to mention his flagrant disregard for safety, never entered my mind. I also didn't weigh in about smoking and the total indifference this man showed for his personal health, especially considering his profession. He ruled this world and I was entranced.

Chaos roiled in front of us like an enraged cobra, hissing and spewing venom, striking again and again. The paramedic, relaxed in the face of absolute frenzy, caressed our speeding ambulance through the streets to arrive at an apartment I mistook for a storage shed.

Inside the one-room house, a man had beaten his wife and continued to verbally assault her with a vicious barrage. The medic strode in and halted the screams of rampant fury. The cops arrived while he tended to the battered woman and told her,

"Leave the guy. You're worth more than this. It's going to get worse. He may even kill you."

He then turned and soothed the anxieties of the frightened children who didn't come up to the height of the gun holsters worn about the room.

I wanted to do that, to take down fear with a cold stare, to pull answers from the drug box I held at my side, to be the reason people said,

"Thanks for helping me."

He was my idol. I wanted to be just like him.

A paramedic.

I started on that road soon after when I moved to Tuscaloosa, Alabama for college and took the class for my EMT certificate. On paper, I knew what to do in an emergency.

Yeah, right.

CHAPTER 4

Chad Rayne

"Are you going to leave that thing on all day?" Chad bellowed, three feet from my right ear, his foot on the ambulance dash. The turn signal lever was broken and I had forgotten to cancel the incessant clicking. Chad continued his verbal rant, yelling to the wind out his open window.

"You're a zero, a zero, a ZERO!"

Chad Rayne, "God," Paramedic. My first partner.

Two weeks before, I had walked up to the first ambulance I hoped to call mine. Inside, Chad moved smoothly from cabinets to boxes while Lucy, his partner, opened and closed doors, arranged items, filling empty spaces. I crawled in to join them, sitting on the bench seat near the back door, scanning the equipment we carried.

Lucy tripped over my feet as she jumped out.

I mumbled, "Sorry," and scooted farther up the bench.

Chad dropped a box next to me and flipped open the lid, hitting me in the arm.

I squeaked out another, "Sorry," moved two inches to the back again, and the first-day barely-contained butterflies in my stomach turned into a bubbling cauldron of lava.

Five minutes ago this ambulance seemed large enough for the three of us to perform our jobs. Now, things spun the other direction and the ambulance was just a van, stripped of its interior and replaced with cabinets bursting with medical items, a good portion of which I didn't recognize. The gurney filled most of the floor space, leaving barely the length of my shoe's distance to the bench where I sat. To top it all off, the "job" I was here to do? Well, I didn't have one. I was just in the way.

Lucy dropped an armload of nasal cannulas on the bench, spilling them against my thigh.

"Here. Put these away."

I anxiously scanned the cabinets, peering through the clear plastic doors, trying to find the home for nasal cannulas. To appear more intense I stood, leaned toward the next cabinet and slid the door open, only to locate a few bandaging supplies. I closed that door and opened the next, where medications in different colored boxes lay side by side. Moving on, my hand brushed needles neatly taped to the walls and ready for instant access. Still further I found packages and bags and bins overflowing. No nasal cannulas.

Lucy's voice floated from behind as I searched.

"Up there, right side, third shelf down."

I peered over Chad, busy with his boxes, and found the hole.

The more I looked, the more scared I became. I had just finished a semester-long EMT class, taken the test, did rather well, graduated, and was authorized — the State said so — to work on an ambulance. Now, inside an actual ambulance, I sat lost in an alien world, a big dolt wearing a nametag to help me remember my own name.

Trying valiantly not to seem like dead wood, I turned to Lucy as she approached with an armload of IV bags.

"Excuse me," I stammered. "In case we get a call . . ."

Lucy hefted the weight of the bags as she stood, waiting, outside the ambulance.

"What should I do?"

"Just follow us." She dropped the bags on the end of the gurney. "Put these away."

Hmm, not very helpful. This was important. I was not going to spend the day like a prom dance wallflower. I found the place for the IV bags and turned to Chad as he checked a box full of supplies. He slid open a drawer, rolled a few tiny bottles around and pushed it back in. The next drawer he pulled out held syringes and he counted those while I stood over his shoulder, still lost and now invisible.

Chad closed that drawer and stuffed his hand into the bottom section to lift out a plastic bag looking like a football with tubing. I recognized it from EMT school as the bag-valve-mask, or BVM, which kept the user from physically doing mouth-to-mouth breathing on a patient. Chad peered into the depths left by removing the BVM. Without looking up he spoke.

"First day on the job, huh?"

"I, um, well, I . . ."

Chad continued, "We'll take good care of you."

"I, ah . . . What should I . . ."

Chad cut me off, saving me from myself.

"You just follow Lucy and me. Grab what we tell you to grab and stay right next to me. If we start to run away, make sure you're in the ambulance first."

He stopped counting, looked at me, pulled half a smile, and went back to work.

Oh God, I thought. *If we run away, make sure I'm in the ambulance first? That was it? That was my orientation?*

Chad was leading me into a place where I could get caught in a fistfight, a stray bullet could kill me, and I could fall through the broken steps. To survive in this world I had to catch every nuance, know everything about my ambulance, and be acutely aware of my surroundings. Ignorance could kill me, my partner, or my patient. In this world, change morphed with deception and stealth. In this world, death came with subtle clues.

Later in the day we got a Code Blue. I had no idea what that was. We arrived and I hopped out, clearing the ambulance like a commando on a mission, the oxygen bottle tucked under my arm, a nasal cannula and oxygen mask bulging from my pockets. Chad and Lucy grabbed the equipment boxes. We formed a triangle, Chad on point, and advanced toward the patient. I was ready.

I was not ready.

A man lay motionless on his back in the driveway. His naked belly cleared his belt and rose like a mountain while, from the nipples up, he was purple. A woman—his wife, I figured—tried to revive him with aggressive compressions to his abdomen. She knew she was supposed to press on something to do the reviving, but wasn't sure exactly what. With her arms pressing up and down, hair swinging back and forth in time with her efforts, she gave it all she had.

Chad ran to the man's side, weighted with equipment. He ripped open packages and attached wires to stickers while Lucy tore through the medical box, pulled out the BVM and began its assembly. I stood behind her, stunned by the whole scene, and watched Chad decide our race had not been fast enough. Death had won.

This wasn't school, chapter five, page one hundred and fifty-three. This was life and I had witnessed the end of one. The wife sat back on the driveway and sobbed. Lucy gathered our equipment and the trash we created in a few frantic minutes. Chad did paperwork and talked into his radio. He turned to me.

"Scott, go get a sheet."

Two weeks later another patient made the mistake of getting out of bed on a warm day without a cloud in the sky. The man had gone for a motorcycle ride in an idyllic neighborhood where kids played ball and dogs romped in the yards. A tree branch snapped off and struck the guy in the chest, ripping him off his bike.

I climbed out of the ambulance next to the bike lying on its side, the sissy bar bent backwards. I followed Chad to the patient. On the guy's chest, bared by firefighters already on the scene, I saw a little dark spot below his left nipple. A sucking chest wound!

Sucking chest wounds are fascinating. Air goes in the wrong hole; pressure builds up; it pushes the lung to the side and doesn't allow it to re-inflate. Luckily, when recognized, they are easy to fix—plug it. To do this, EMT class instructed us to use a 4x4-inch piece of gauze impregnated with petroleum jelly as a dressing. My school text directed us to carefully lay the gauze over the hole, maintaining sterility of the dressing against the skin by never touching the underside during removal from the package. We had been instructed to place tape on three sides to allow air to escape the wrongly pressurized chest cavity but not permit new air to enter.

Chad knelt and started his assessment of the chest. There isn't much tissue on this part of the body and this simple-looking wound, a hole really, led between the ribs smack into the heart, lungs, and blood vessels. Being a medic made Chad privy to the big stuff. In fact, he was called to come and inspect it.

I took up my position at the guy's left shoulder while Lucy chatted it up with the cops. (I suspect this is what moved me up to actual partner, promoted from voluntary ride-along).

Chad asked for the petroleum gauze. I flipped open the box I brought to the patient, slipped my hand down the right side of the bottom section, pulled out the silver package and handed it to him.

Chad grasped the flaps at the top of the package firmly, peeling open the foil wrapper. After exposing the gauze, he pinched the upper surface precisely at the middle, removing it from the foil while maintaining sterility. Chad's precision as he followed the exact technique we had been taught thrilled me. Then he threw the gauze over his left shoulder and applied the foil wrapper, not the gauze, to the wound.

Afterward, Chad explained.

"The inside of the package is sterile, tape sticks better to the foil and is less messy than spreading that gooey shit everywhere."

My partner truly was Chad Rayne, "God," Paramedic.

Actually, that *is* what he called himself.

He would pose in the middle of dispatch, chin jutting to the right, frozen in hero posture, and announce his name using his deepest resonating voice, chest puffed out and hands on his hips, an imaginary cape fluttering behind.

"Chad Rayne, *God*, Paramedic!"

Hold… and cue the tooth sparkle.

Overblown? Sure. But, that was Chad. Young, good looking, with a trim body and a strong jaw, his gaze burnt through to my soul or melted the heart of a new and pretty nurse before he walked out with her phone number.

He was brash, swaggering, hilarious, and disrespectful. During our time together, Chad glued quarters to desks, thumb-tacked pizza slices to the door and called the phone booth seen from the office's tinted window. No one was safe from his antics. Once he dragged a young female co-worker outside, held her by the arm, and yelled for the whole neighborhood to hear,

"White woman for sale!"

We also worked ourselves silly. Our shifts were twenty-four hours on, forty-eight hours off. We got paid four dollars an hour for twenty out of twenty-four hours. The company had used a loophole and found our jobs were classed, federally, as interstate truckers. Management didn't have to pay us the full twenty-four hours.

Despite his antics, Chad was the paramedic I wanted to become. We walked into strangers' houses like we'd been there before. Once inside, Chad's word was law. The TV got turned off, all smokers either put out the butts or left the room, and family members remained available for questioning. The fish in the aquarium didn't hide behind a rock without checking with Chad.

But that presence being thrown about had a downside: Chad had better deliver. He accepted the challenge by walking in the door. He was fast to catch why the lady was short of breath and he was thorough to find the bullet hole in the boy's armpit. In the ambulance, he beat back Death while standing up without a seatbelt at seventy miles an hour. He also had to tolerate me.

I drove to the hospital with a patient at three o'clock in the morning for some minor complaint. I didn't see the speed bump. The explosion to the front wheels and then the back sounded like I tore the chassis from the body of the ambulance. Neither Chad, nor the patient, said anything. Even at the hospital, Chad didn't yell, scream, or give me a nasty look as I pulled the gurney from the ambulance.

After completing the paperwork, we got back in the ambulance. Chad caught my eye, held the gaze for a few seconds, then dramatically tossed himself, arms flailing, rocking the ambulance with his efforts, all over the seat and about the cab. It was clearly a re-creation of his end of the experience with the speed bump.

Soon, there were two of us on the ambulance, no longer three, and we had an auto accident outside of town. After loading the patient, Chad said, "Okay, you know how to blow intersections. Drive as fast as you feel safe."

In quieter moments, Chad used to point to the patch sewn on the shoulder of his uniform, a Nationally Registered Paramedic patch. Stitched with blue and gold metallic thread, it glittered.

As he pointed, he would repeat a phrase pulled from an old ad run by the Yamaha motorcycle company. "One of these days you'll own a Yamaha."

I knew what he meant: One of these days you'll be a paramedic and you'll be permitted to put one of these on your uniform.

Hey, Chad. I'm wearing one. I own a Yamaha.

Thanks, Chad.

CHAPTER 5

Kissing A Dead Guy

"No, sir. We do not give a death discount." Rachel, the Notre Dame of Administration, faced the man standing at the collection window of the ambulance company, bill in hand. He attempted to make his case as Ted, my partner with Chad on vacation, and I stepped past him on our way out of the office en route to a motorcycle accident.

He obviously began to protest because Rachel offered Statement Number Two.

"Yes, sir. I realize the bill is rather unsettling." Rachel countered his next parry.

"I'm sorry, sir. But this is what is involved in having our paramedics try to save your loved one. I am sorry for your loss."

Ted pushed on the glass door and we entered the realm of the July Alabama sun, leaving Rachel to bring the man down kindly. Practice makes perfect.

Even though I'd been in Alabama for nearly a year and doing this job for two months, the sun still surprised me. They left that part out of the travel brochure. Oh, there'd been mention of the Sunny South. But they failed to use the proper adjectives when describing the summer months in that *Sunny South*. It was freaking hot. The only saving grace? Air conditioning. Without that, this Yankee would have scampered back to north of the Mason-Dixon Line. My pores didn't work that hard.

I stepped outside and the heat slammed into my face, then seared my lungs with the first breath. Sunglasses saved my eyes but already the plastic of the nosepiece cooked into my skin. At the ambulance I hazarded second-degree burns to pop open the door handle.

Inside the cab, even the air sweated and, in contact with the seat, my polyester pants began to melt. The ignition scalded my fingers, a necessity to achieve the relief of air conditioning.

The starter was rough, but I knew the secret: Let her roll and grind three times, then stomp the accelerator to the floor. I flipped the toggle switches for the emergency lights, turned on the siren, and threw the gearshift into drive while scorching my palm. I accelerated, turning left as fast as the old goat would allow. Ted, buckled up, placed his right foot on the dash.

Betty in Dispatch had sent us to Highway 345 at the strip mines, a local piece of dirt beloved by the off-roaders because the mining company took off the top layer of soil, removed everything of value, and left. She said to watch for the guy's brother, he would lead us in.

He began as a speck on the side of the road. As we got closer, the speck became a young man on a dirt bike waving in frantic arcs over his head.

Ted made an astute observation.

"Must be the brother."

We closed the gap, but before Ted took his foot off the dash the guy stopped waving, grabbed the handlebars, squirted across the road and down a dirt track to disappear among the pines.

Ted made another helpful observation.

"Better follow him. Don't want to lose him."

I slowed and turned left into a split between the trees where dirt still settled back to the trail.

"I'll follow the dust," I said, beating Ted to the punch.

The narrow path dipped and crawled as branches scraped down the sides of the ambulance. I tried to avoid a few of the larger craters while keeping an eye out for overhangs. Ripping the light bar off the top wouldn't be good. The fire department in their ambulance followed, their lights flashing through our billowing wake. We escaped the trees to enter a barren landscape where dirt hills, sparse with scrawny shrubs, rolled to meet the sky.

The biker sat far ahead of us on a rise, again beckoning with wild swings of his arms.

I spoke, as if he could hear me.

"We're coming. We're coming. I can't move this thing any faster. Oof!"

A large pothole punctuated the last word and my head tossed left, almost into the window next to me. Ted took his foot off the dash.

We started up the rise as the biker sped off again down the other side.

"How am I supposed to keep up with this guy?" I said, more to myself than anybody.

I was done getting beaten up by the lack of sensible road, following someone on a dirt bike using an overstocked van.

As I came toward the crest, Ted said firmly, "Stop."

I stomped the brake and slid in the dirt.

Ted continued.

"Don't go over the hill. We'll high-center on top."

What is 'high-center?' Never heard of that before.

I thought a moment. If I drove the front wheels over the ridge, the bottom of the ambulance would get hung up before the rear wheels cleared the peak. We would be teetering with the center of the chassis on the dirt and none of the wheels on the ground.

"Put it in park, let's get out."

I followed Ted's direction and got out. The fire department guys did the same.

Everybody met at the back of the ambulance and, as a group, we all stared at the top of the rise. The biker was further off into the wasteland. Maybe by collective effort we could make him come back.

Didn't work.

This was insane and not like the clean emergency calls I experienced so far. Up until now we stepped out of the ambulance, grabbed our boxes and equipment, went into the house, and promptly located the patient because a loving family member showed us the way. Today, our only possibility of finding the injured person had ridden over a dirt hill and left us. Even worse, none of the others standing with me appeared concerned or even surprised.

One of the firefighters spoke.

"Well, I guess we start grabbing shit."

I took this to mean we were walking.

Everybody grabbed some necessary item. Ted hoisted the medical box, a brown and tan fishing tackle box converted to our most-used kit. Both pursuits needed little trays to put a small collection of stuff in, and this model's two tiers folded up and back when the lid opened. An expanse in the bottom held everything else. The box contained medicines, IV lines, needles, and the BVM. I stepped forward to receive my implement and got leftovers: The backboard, a six-foot length of plywood used to secure someone who might have a neck or back injury.

I grabbed the board by the hand-hold on the side. Finding the board's center, I tested the optimum carry method to not hit me in the legs while running. Finished, I scanned our party to confirm our readiness and continue our rush to the patient.

No one ran.

What?

We couldn't drive any farther, requiring us to walk, and everybody around me, except our lost biker guy, seemed off to a Sunday meeting. Out in the sun and dirt someone needed our help and seconds could make the difference.

Hurry, damn it!

I ran to the top of the hill, my backboard swinging and hitting the dirt. From the crest I peered through the heated and undulating air rising over a monotonous landscape of red clay, with shrubs dotting the ground. About half a mile across the scrub, the biker leaned down next to a shape.

His brother.

I ran down the hill, trying to keep the backboard from digging in and sending me cart-wheeling the rest of the way. In the valley between hills I lost sight of the patient, but I had plotted a path across the moonscape. The bushes slid past, the board slapping some and missing others.

My new black boots became covered in fine red dust. Steel-toed, they weren't this heavy since the first time I put them on. Now, apparently, even the leather turned to lead. I refocused to dodge more bushes, missed and tripped, stumbled and kept going, rewarded with a face full of dust.

The sun was back. The punishing orb never left, but the excitement blocked my senses. Now I fully realized I was running through a deserted wasteland, wearing heavy boots, a full uniform of clothing and carrying a slab of plywood in mid-summer. Sweat cascaded from every available source. With each breath the torrent around my mouth got sucked in and blown out in a spray. Only three things lived out here: dirt, bushes, and sky. My backboard and I did not blend with the environment. I tripped over more shrubbery to find the dirt spiced the same as before: with essence of grit.

I crested the hill and a few yards down the other side the man cradled his fallen brother. Two dirt bikes lay nearby like discarded toys. I stumbled over, throwing the backboard to the side, breathing hard.

I had arrived. Called to an emergency, I overcame several obstacles to get here. I even grabbed a medical device, my backboard, and physically ran to where I couldn't drive. I suffered a lot. About then I short-circuited.

What lay before me, covered in dust and blood, up until now, could only be referenced in Chapter 3, pages 63-84, albeit in color photography. According to that chapter, my job entailed curing the sick and injured. What exactly did that mean? I didn't have my text at the moment and I'm sure this was mentioned in the Summary section.

I stood over a real person. A little blood mixed with dirt smeared his face. His helmet lay nearby, seemingly removed, because the rest of him still wore all the gear expected for dirt-biking.

The brother looked up at me, his eyes screaming desperation. He had seen his brother fall and knew there were serious injuries. Doing all he could, he rode out of the strip mine, found a phone, called the people who could help, and led them back to where his brother lay in the dirt and the hot sun.

I was "the people." Me, the one with two months of experience and a lousy chunk of plywood for company. The brother waited. Either it was time to start making origami or I had better do something.

I dropped to my knees and scrutinized the face of a young man no older than me, twenty at most. He slept. That's what unconsciousness looked like.

Unconsciousness! That was important.

Back in my CPR course a mannequin lay in front of me and the steps for saving a life scrolled in my brain.

Step number one: Shake the patient and shout, "Annie, Annie! Are you okay?"

I reached out and shook the man lying in the dirt. No response. He was now officially unconscious.

I moved on to step number two: Look, listen, and feel. I remembered the focus of this step involved opening his mouth to check for breathing. However, there was a caveat. If the incident involved trauma, I must open his mouth but prevent movement of his neck using a special maneuver in case it was broken. I quickly categorized a motorcycle accident causing unconsciousness as having the possibility to break a neck and most probably fit the bill for trauma. I was to use this maneuver.

I moved around to the top of his head so I could open his mouth, lifting on both sides of his jaw. That done, I put my ear near his mouth, listened for breathing and twisted my neck around to confirm his chest did not rise. I also did not feel any of his breath on my cheek. He was not breathing, officially.

On to step number three. I must move rapidly giving the patient the best chance for survival; seconds meant the difference. I shifted back, next to his shoulder, tripped over my boots in my haste, and kicked up dirt on the way.

A dusty layer settled on my patient's face. That wasn't nice and not mentioned in the book. I was supposed to be helping him and I made him dirtier.

Stop. Focus. Step number three.

Step number three was the commitment step. According to the book, steps one and two confirmed my patient was indeed having an emergency and required life-saving breathing. Step number three was next. About this point there would be no quarreling. I read it in the book.

I opened the man's mouth and pinched his nose closed to prevent air escaping. I lowered my mouth to his and blew all my air into his body. I pulled back an inch or two and took another breath releasing it once again into his lungs. His clothes rose over his chest.

I did it! I breathed two life-saving breaths into another person's lungs. Step number three! I did step number three on a real person!

Step number four. I placed two fingers on his neck, searching for his carotid pulse. My fingers, dripping with sweat, slid out of the depression, leaving a muddy streak. I put them back and held firm for several seconds. Nothing. No pulse. This meant swiftly invoking step number five and beginning compressions on his chest, one and a half to two inches in depth, to compress the heart between the breast bone and the spine. This action squeezed the heart, forcing the blood out and around the body, then back to complete the circuit. My continued breathing for him put oxygen in that blood and I would save his life.

I shifted slightly and placed my hands in the proper position on his breastbone, one over the other, and pressed vigorously down, then up, down and up, down and up. I did this fifteen times. I moved back to his head, opened his mouth, pinched his nose and gave him two more breaths.

When I came up from the second breath I had, by now, left enough sweat and saliva behind and this was no longer a dry procedure. With moisture came taste. I began another round of chest compressions while sampling an interesting mixture of flavors then mentally separated each one.

Let's see, that one is blood. It was kind of sweet.

That one must be his saliva.

I had reached number four on the second round of compressions when everything went from a huge swirl and blur to zip into absolute clarity.

This is disgusting!

I am blowing into some guy's mouth to whom, by the way, I have never been formally introduced. I am sampling his blood while mixing my sweat with his spit and finishing with a big gargle of the whole concoction.

Someone forgot to write this section in the book.

A cynical light bulb went on. No, no one forgot. It was intentionally left out. They published the sterile version, the cleaned up scenario. If the truth were written, there would be no takers. I had been betrayed.

Yuck!

I kept count of my chest compressions with a mumble. "Seven, eight, nine, ten."

In just five more ups and downs I was headed back for another dose. The nausea twisted in my stomach.

"Fourteen, fifteen."

Damn, here I go.

My lips to his lips. Blow and blow. Back to the chest.

Oh, this is gross. How long am I supposed to keep this up?

I again referred to the book. After the flowery description filled with heroic instruction, yes, a mention had been made of when to stop:

Once one entered into the grand decision to cheat death of another victim, one could stop CPR when instructed to do so by a medical professional of higher authority or when too exhausted to continue.

There was no gross-out clause.

Shit.

I was young, fit, in the geographic center of freakin' Sahara Desert, Alabama, not a doctor in sight and had just begun. I was locked in. Doomed. My destiny until the next whenever was to swap spit with some dead guy.

I settled into a morose calm about the whole situation.

Five, six, seven, eight . . . .

"Stop. Scott, just stop."

A hand rested on my shoulder and stayed in time with my up and down bobbing of chest compressions.

"You can stop, Scott. You don't have to do this."

Ted finally arrived with his brown tackle box in tow, the one with the bag-valve-mask. Those three words succinctly described its parts: Bag, valve, and mask. There was the bag, the size of a football, which the rescuer compressed to force sweet, life-giving air through the valve. Once through this valve, the air swirled majestically into the mask and over the patient's face while the rescuer kept his own mouth a discrete three feet away. The air completed its trip and mission by arriving in the non-breathing person's lungs. It was like mouth-to-mouth — only better.

I sat back in the dirt and closed my eyes. The sun made the view of my eyelids a muted yellow while the sweat formed a solid stream down my face. I breathed the air and pondered again all the flavors of my experience.

Ted said quietly, "What were you doing?"

The question sent a needle into my balloon of confidence and I answered with a voice like a question mark.

"He didn't have a pulse. He wasn't breathing. I did CPR."

Ted's voice again came over my shoulder.

"Didn't you see the ants and brains coming out of his ears?"

I leaned over the far side of his head from where I knelt. A simple line of black ants marched silently over a mass of gray porridge.

My glorious moment turned black in half a second. My head went into a swirl again as my thoughts pleaded for something to hold.

What have I done?

I had done mouth-to-mouth on a guy that didn't need it. Well, he did, but it wouldn't work. I failed and, to make things worse, a foul swill of flavors inhabited my mouth to provide an underscore I would retain forever.

Only doing the job two months, I had been out in front on this one. I ran to a patient's side, reached into the bag containing limited experience, and pulled out an assessment followed by a plan of action. But it was wrong.

The forensic sample I collected was not a badge of honor for performing the ultimate personal life-saving measure. I shared saliva with a dead guy because I hadn't done a thorough exam. I was not to be the recipient of congratulations for being new to the business and daring to be aggressive. I was to be the subject of giggling discussion around the water cooler.

I needed a toothbrush.

I rose out of the dirt and stepped into the bushes while the sun continued to wash my body in sweat. The t-shirt under my uniform, being soaking wet, chilled my back as I walked, which contrasted nicely from my face. I stopped and spit out any collection of saliva gathering in my mouth.

Behind me a small knot of observers stood over the freshly dead. The brother sat in the dirt and curled himself around one knee, holding on tightly as the sobs racked his back. Ted spoke into the radio he brought with him. I wandered toward the group to find out the next step.

When I arrived, the firefighters had the courtesy not to drag me through any more hell. They could see my disgust. But I knew they only filed me away until they got back to their station. I was to be tonight's roast during dinner.

Ted smiled kindly.

"Betty already called a helicopter to airlift this guy to the hospital. Once they spin up those rotors the big money is spent. I told her we can use them to at least get our patient back to the ambulance. We're here until they show up."

Everybody peeled off in different directions. The firefighters stepped a few feet into the bushes to walk the boundary between private conversation and being near enough to appear interested. Ted, the paramedic in charge of this scene, still had paperwork to do and information to gather from the grieving brother.

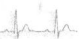

I'm not sure where they came from with no houses to be seen, no road visible. Two of them, two girls about eighteen or nineteen, sauntered across the scrabble of dirt and rocks. My confusion about their origin became overwhelmed by amazement as they walked through the toasty land barefoot.

They wore t-shirts and cut-off jeans, both of which left too much of themselves in other places. One, a brunette, led the way. Her hair, falling below her shoulders, swayed a little as she walked around a bush. A blonde followed. They slowed as they approached.

"Hey, what y'all doing?" said the brunette, her voice sweet and soft. Then she saw our guy under the bush. "Ew, what happened to him?"

"He wrecked on his motorcycle. Killed himself," I said.

She puffed her lower lip out.

"I'm sorry for that. I hope it didn't hurt."

I didn't know.

"No, if he hit real hard, it probably killed him right off."

"So, what y'all doing here," asked the blonde. "What ya going to do with him?"

"Waiting on a helicopter. We're going to fly him out."

Her eyes shot wide and a grin flashed on her face.

"A helicopter? Oh, that'll be neat."

The carnival was coming to town.

"Can we stay till it gets here? I ain't never seen a helicopter up close."

I thought about it. I could ask them to leave but who was I to tell them where to go? She and her friend would just walk off a short distance, stand somewhere else and be even be more trouble when the helicopter came.

"Yeah, you can stay. But you have to be careful and stay out of the way."

They both giggled. The brunette turned to her friend and then back.

"We'll be good. We promise. We'll do whatever you say."

That settled, we were now left to wait.

We all stood in the dirt with two bored firefighters sort of nearby while Ted cradled a clipboard and shuffled back and forth between my personal friend, the dead guy, and his grieving brother. While I stood under a blazing sun, losing a quart of water an hour into my boots, two scruffy girls kept us company while looking increasingly like my imaginings about backwoods Southern women.

They were not from the sultry, sexy, Southern women classification I had filed away. These two were more of the "Deliverance" category: Quite attractive women who carried an air suggesting danger from shotgun-toting male relatives. It was all a stereotype, I knew, but I had no interest in testing the theory.

My problem was multi-layered. The foul assemblage of my new buddy swam with prominence in my mouth, resisting the fall toward dehydration, while my boots birthed the environment for trench foot, filling with expunged sweat. No helicopter spun from the horizon while the Deliverance twins showed up on an afternoon stroll from nowhere, comfortably barefoot on Mother Nature's griddle, chatting it up while standing over a fresh dead guy lying in the bushes. Was this normal? Were they used to this sort of thing?

The brunette sidled up a little closer.

"Do you guys work a lot?"

I had to think about this. Conversation didn't seem proper while I watched over a dead body. I didn't see any invading armies coming to lay claim. But, it felt unacceptable to be social at a time like this. I also couldn't be rude.

"Yeah, we work twenty-four hour shifts."

Keep the answers short, they might get bored and go away.

"Twenty-four hours. Oh, my." Her mouth opened in overdone surprise. "Don't you ever get tired?"

"We're allowed to sleep when we're not on a call."

Short answers. Keep it polite and professional but don't encourage. She was cute but this was just too weird.

"So, what ya doing after work? Would you like to go out and have a drink?"

That did it. I flipped into surreal overload. I stood not more than ten feet from a dead guy I had just kissed. His brains, no longer neatly encased in his skull, had ants making them a parade ground. Five of us live ones, now seven adding Trixie and Dixie here, all stood in the sweltering heat watching the dead guy and waiting with our thumbs stuck out for a passing helicopter to take us back to Kansas. I was clicking my heels real hard while getting asked out on a date.

I stammered my response.

"I, um, I work a lot and I also go to school." It was actually all true. Besides my full-time shifts on the ambulance, I was going to class, attending my hospital rotations, and doing ride-alongs with Tuscaloosa Fire to get my EMT-Level II certificate. "But thank you for asking."

The brunette slumped a little but gave me a sideways glance clearly stating the offer still stood. I smiled weakly, knowing I wouldn't be asking for her phone number.

I moved closer to my latest patient, feeling like someone should keep him company. The nearby feeble branches of a dried up bush supplied his only protection as he slowly baked in the sun. He stared without blinking into the unbroken blue sky. Some thoughts rambled through my head.

I can't stare into the sun like that. I would have to blink.

My mother always said, "Never stare into the sun, you'll go blind."

I didn't know what was proper. Should I cover his face? Was I allowed to disturb the body? Did it matter or was I trying to make myself feel better?

He appeared quite serene and seemed, at any moment, about to breathe. I waited, then realized I was waiting and told myself, no, that would never happen. This man died and this was what death looked like. Nothing. What made him alive, what energized his eyes, his skin, his muscles, had gone. He was now a fleshy shell roasting in the sun.

He and his brother got up this morning and decided to go for a motorcycle ride. He had a date tonight or something different for dinner. Maybe not. Maybe this was going to be another night watching television. It didn't matter.

I turned to look for his tire tracks. I searched the dust for the imprint, the clue to his final half-second of sensibility. I wanted to find the moment where things horribly changed. I walked slowly back and forth at the crest of the hill. Footprints and tire tracks muddied the signs.

If I found the tracks perhaps I could find the rock that changed the course of the day for so many people. There must be blood or a scuff mark, a burrow in the dirt or something. This man could not have died without leaving a sensible trail to tell the story. A path had to exist leading up to where he now lay. I wanted to follow that path and make a logical conclusion that the body dead before me followed the laws of physics and, if one performed the same trail of events, the same outcome would occur. I wanted to make sense of it.

Not this time. People died. People died and they didn't leave a pretty path to make the living feel better. The dirt was dirt, the rocks simply rocks. They all lay about in their haphazard fashion, as they always did, none offering up the other as the perpetrator in a man's death.

CHAPTER 6

Scrawny Bryan

Part-time work on an ambulance in college was the best job ever. For three years, I'd walk into the manager's office in May and say, "I'm finished with finals on the sixteenth."

"Fantastic! I'll hire you full-time."

In August I'd again walk into the manager's office.

"My classes start the twenty-sixth."

"Okay, we'll drop you back to part-time."

For the next eight months my phone would ring.

"Yeah, um, Scott? Can you work Saturday?"

"Well . . . no. I've got a date Saturday. I can work Sunday, though."

"Fantastic! We've got a shift then, too."

Come May, "My finals are over the twenty-first."

Best job ever!

Not that I was doing it the right way. Finished with my freshman year of college, and on summer break, I worked full time and was having the time of my life. I barely knew how to be an EMT, much less a good one, but I asked my coworkers, "So, what's next?"

They told me I should take the class for the next level of EMT. I did, and by the end of summer I had advanced to EMT-Intermediate.

"Hey guys, what's next?"

"Now you go to paramedic school."

They offered that at the university, too. I signed up and soon finished. One year and three months after touching my first ambulance I was a paramedic, twenty years old, walking into people's houses and expected to save their life from whatever mess they had gotten themselves into.

In August I also signed up for fall semester classes. The first class I always put down was marching band. I applied to Ohio State and the University of Alabama because they both had famous marching bands. With my dad living in Alabama, I qualified for in-state fees (cheaper) and still moved away from home. Not that I didn't like home. It just wasn't somewhere else.

I knew all I wanted out of college was something to augment being a paramedic. I figured a biology major would do. Beyond that I was there for the marching band. Some of my best memories of college are from the band: The road trips, the away games.

They sent 360 of us band students to New York City my freshman year for the Kick-off Classic. Over the next five years I made it to El Paso, Texas; New Orleans, Louisiana; Tampa, Florida; and Disney World. Well, Disney World lacked a bit. We marched around that place and played the fight song thirty times. Afterward we gathered, and the director told us, "Okay, you can go into Epcot Center for free. We'll see you back here in . . . four hours."

After one ride and a meal we were done. Woo hoo!

I was also in a fraternity, which, in Alabama, is another dimension. I, however, couldn't stomach the whole concept and gladly joined TKE. They fit my style, had parties, but didn't get hung up in all the stuffiness. Some folks say, "If you can't go Greek, go Teke." Well, looking back, I'd say, "Boys, get over yourselves."

I don't drink alcohol. I don't like the taste, nothing fancier than that. I spent my time at the parties honing a new craft. We had one musician come by frequently. Russ Rosser was a one-man band and simply phenomenal. He played guitar and sang, ran his own mixing board and a drum machine. The best part was the bass guitar. He re-tooled a bass, put it on the floor, and played by pressing pedals with his feet.

At one of the parties I summoned the gumption to sit in and play improvisational saxophone. This meant he told me a few details about the mechanics of the song and off we went. I made stuff up and tried to make it fit. Background, solos, he even let me sing. If I became stubborn or tried something completely off, he shut down my microphone. We had an understanding. After a while, Russ started inviting me to play gigs with him around town. I'm not sure how well I played at the time because some years later, with another group, a talented musician said he had been talking to another band member. "Scott sure sounds good, but he has no idea what he's doing."

But that was in my off-duty time. On-duty I was in a different world.

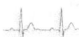

I bolted from my seat, lunging at the hand my patient had freed from his restraints. His piercing scream acted as its own assault as he strained for the needles taped to the wall.

"Hey, John! Pull over. I need help!"

I grabbed the flailing arm at the moment he freed his second hand, which struggled to find the seat belt release. We wrestled our way down the freeway as I held him to the gurney in a headlock.

"John! Pull Over!"

I met Bryan only an hour before, as he was led out of the holding cell in Tuscaloosa's brand spanking new jail. What he was there for I didn't know and didn't particularly care. They released him to me so his crime must not have been that bad. My partner, John, and I were charged with taking Bryan to a psychiatric facility in northeast Georgia, a six-hour drive. Management dictated we put the patient in restraints. Bryan was not large, just a scrawny kid of eighteen, and we faced a long ride.

I approached him, holding lightweight, cloth restraints.

"Sorry, just following orders."

Bryan smiled but said nothing. He offered his arms for the procedure.

Bryan spent the first hour of the trip educating me on how to maintain a quality high with the proper use of ether.

"Ether by itself is horrible. It makes you drunk but your legs shake and you're scared. Totally sucks. You have to mix it with a gas, like carbon dioxide. Then your whole body is spinning but you're not even dizzy."

He seemed to think on this for a while, reliving the memory, before he continued.

"Mixed with ethylene it's even better. I didn't feel a thing when I got poked with a knife."

Bryan fidgeted and he strained against the ties holding his hands as he related more of his experience with ether.

"My friend dug into me and I didn't feel nothing. To make the ethylene, I took alcohol and sulfuric acid. I mixed them at 175 degrees."

Bryan still tried to use his hands to talk but they stopped short every time due to the ties. His eyes were bright and animated and, while he told his spirited story, he practically hopped on the gurney, held down only by two seat belts and his restrained arms.

"It has to be 175 degrees. Can't be cooler than that."

I didn't imagine myself using this information in the near future but it was interesting how detailed he was in his knowledge. I also was not sure where he got the ether because I didn't think surgeons used it anymore. Maybe he was making all this up. Oh, well, I stayed awake and he seemed to enjoy the topic, judging by how much he jumped around. Bryan had a hobby and I continued to listen.

Then one hand pulled free and grabbed toward the needles on the wall. Now he and I wrestled to see who would keep whom inside the ambulance while on the freeway. John whipped to the side of the road, then jumped in back and joined the fracas.

I yelled, "Sit on him. He's almost got that seat belt figured out." I held Bryan's head and avoided his clawing fingers as they searched for me behind the gurney. "Watch out. His left hand is free."

John grabbed the wayward hand, dodged a few kicks and dropped his weight on Bryan's legs.

"Little shit tried to kick me in the balls."

John adjusted his grip on the boy's wrist, then gave me directions.

"Got his hand. Grab that other one. Come around to the front. Sit on him. I'll grab some sheets. Tie his ass down."

I was sweaty; so was Bryan as he fought with everything he had. Firmly holding his right hand and shifting to put an elbow in his chest, I walked myself around to his front. Bryan pulled loose in the process.

"Damn. I lost his hand!"

A barrage of fingers and pinches, like a swarm of attacking locusts, held me back until I drove my knee into his chest and grabbed both of his arms.

Bryan's head, with teeth bared, came shooting forward. I twisted away and shoved my forearm under his chin, pushing his throat back to the gurney.

"Sucker tried to bite me."

Bryan's hands slipped free again from my sweaty grip. I ducked and lay on top of him using my left arm to block his fists and my right hand to grab a hunk of hair. Bryan screamed in my ear.

I yelled, "Okay. I think I have him. Get some sheets."

John's weight rose and Bryan found new purpose in his wriggling. He squirmed down the gurney from under me.

"Hurry with those sheets, John. I can't hold him."

Bryan kicked the back door of the ambulance.

John grabbed his legs, staying clear of the swinging feet, and again gave me directions.

"Okay, get off him, grab his arms, and we'll pull him back up the gurney."

Quickly shifting to the left, I got above Bryan's head and pulled both arms, drawing his body up the bed. Bryan twisted his body and rose from the mattress. I countered by grabbing his hair and pulling him back down but this let an arm free. I dodged again as it swung behind.

"Right arm's free."

"Shit! He's got my hair!" yelled John.

I dug a finger into the angle of Bryan's jaw near his ear and spoke with malice.

"Let go!"

Bryan screamed in pain and released John's hair to search for my hand digging into his neck, slowing his attack for a moment.

I took advantage of the lull to release a lever, dropping the head of the gurney flat. In a flash, I swung around to Bryan's front, stuck a knee on his chest, and folded myself down on both of his arms with one of my forearms shoving his chin up and pinning his head to the gurney.

"Okay. Got him for a second. Tie one of those sheets around him."

John started wrapping ropes of sheets up Bryan's scrawny body. By the time we finished, and after Bryan got in a few more strikes, four sheets held him to the gurney. But his flailing and pinching hands were still a problem. An ambulance is only so big and sitting on the bench still left me in range. We solved that by gauzing his hands and tying them to the railing. He kept biting at us so we tied two sheets to form an X across his chest, holding him even tighter. He kept kicking the wall of the ambulance so we tied his feet to the left side of the gurney. An hour and a half later we were all a sweaty mess but we had Bryan sealed and under control. All he could do was raise his head.

During the wrestling match, pinpricks of blood had broken out on Bryan's arms. He was coming down from a drug high injected while in that new prison, open for less than a week.

It was my turn to drive, thank God. I crawled in, sank into the seat, breathed deep, and sat, my eyes closed.

"Whew! What a fight."

John heard me.

"Yeah. I'm exhausted. He nearly yanked my hair out. My head *still* hurts."

I had lost my grip on Bryan's hand for that to happen.

"Sorry. He got away from me when we both got sweaty."

"No problem. Get this bus moving. I don't want to spend all day back here."

I put us back on the freeway, still pointed toward Georgia. We hit our cruising speed and Bryan added to the ambiance with the occasional blood-curdling scream. I passed John his set of headphones we usually use to dull the siren noise. Five hours to go.

"Let me go, you monsters!"

Ugh.

"You will die!"

Eventually, Bryan varied his routine. His voice now buttery.

"Let me go. I am the Lord Jesus. Why would you treat Jesus in this manner?"

A few minutes later Bryan got a promotion. His voice reflected his new rank, booming about the ambulance.

"I am God! I will smite thee and bring horrors upon thy children!"

Over the next hour Bryan screamed while becoming or visualizing several gods and prophets.

"I am the Devil! You will pay with your life!"

Bryan had impressive depth of spiritual knowledge.

"I call on the powers of Quetzalcoatl to free me from these bonds!"

After a while he tired and in a plaintive howl he begged, "Please, God. Just give me two bullets to kill the demons! I just need two!"

John and I had switched positions so one demon tried to read a book while John, the other demon, drove us further on this highway to Hell.

Six hours is a long drive.

"Hey John, I'm getting hungry."

"Yeah, me too. There's a town coming up. I'm sure we can find something."

McDonald's worked. No, we did not go through the drive-through with screaming Bryan. At least *we* showed some decorum.

John and I bought him a hamburger, fries, and a shake. With Bryan tucked away in the manner befitting his behavior, he was unable to eat. I had to feed him. We made it about halfway through the hamburger when Bryan tried to bite my hand. The milkshake? What does any child do with a milkshake and a straw? Yeah, he blew into it. Hard. Lunch was over.

As we neared our destination I was driving and John took a look at Bryan.

"Hey, Scott. We can't bring him in trussed up like this."

Bryan was being cooperative and talking to John in a calm voice. I pulled off in a parking lot and crawled in back.

John and I discussed our strategy, inches from the mummified Bryan.

I said, "I'm not untying him all the way."

"No way," said John. "I'm not going through that wrestling match again."

"So, we've got to untie him to make him look better but leave him tied up enough to keep him on the gurney."

No one asked Bryan.

We removed the sheets forming an X on his chest and took off the four holding him to the gurney. We untied his feet from the side but left them restrained separately. Unwrapping the gauze sealing his hands was a smart move. They were red and needed time to relax. We still had them restrained, though. No longer mummy-wrapped, at least they returned to a normal color. Bryan remained calm.

I pulled into the facility, got out, and walked in to the front desk. The place oozed money. The plush carpet silenced all noise from the plod of my steel-toed boots while the light falling from the table lamps to pillowed couches dripped cash.

A nurse looked up as I approached.

"Hi, we're from Tuscaloosa, Alabama. We've got Bryan Jenkins with us. Where do you want him?"

The nurse smiled and said, "Oh, just bring him in here."

"No, ma'am. I don't think you understand. He's been a little . . ." I stopped, searching for the best word, ". . . inappropriate. We really shouldn't wheel him through here."

Her veneer never cracked, "Ah, yes." And she rose from behind her desk to walk outside with me.

She and I stood at the back of the ambulance. Bryan was still strapped to the gurney with seat belts and his arms and feet restrained.

The nurse still held her smile.

"Hi, Bryan. Welcome back."

I'd never considered this could possibly be a return trip.

She continued, "Bryan, are you going to be good if we take off the restraints?"

Bryan was very chipper.

"Yes, ma'am. Nice to see you again, Nurse Dellaport."

"Okay, let him loose."

My heart skipped a beat and I flashed back to the hour and a half spent on the freeway. I didn't want to repeat it. We had, however, just made a transfer of care. Bryan was Nurse Dellaport's charge now. He could leap from the ambulance straight into traffic and nothing would stick to us.

We undid the restraints.

Bryan slid easily off the gurney. I tensed and placed myself between him and the widest path of escape. I could tackle him and John would be right on top of both of us. Bryan and the nurse walked together, arm in arm, into the psych facility and to his room.

I looked at John and we both shook our heads.

John had finished the paperwork before we had pulled in. We spent the next few minutes chatting with the clerk, asking questions about the place and generally stretching our legs.

The nurse came back. I handed her the paperwork and gave my verbal report of the events during transport until another staff member came out and interrupted in a calm voice.

"Excuse me, Nurse Dellaport. Bryan just tried to jump out his window."

CHAPTER 7

Keep 'Em In Stitches

A man calls 911 because he can't get off the floor. We find him in his closet, next to his toolbox. He can't stand up because he's too drunk.

"Sir, what are you doing in the closet?"

"I need some pliers."

"Why do you need pliers?"

"I can't get the top off my beer."

Humor is what gets us through this job. Decisions must be made quickly and decisively with little tolerance for error. We show caring and empathy while we heft the patient down four flights of stairs as he explains how the smelly, week-old leg infection became an emergency at two in the morning. Afterward we write a chart able to withstand legal scrutiny three years later when the case gets to court. Exhausted, we go to sleep on the gurney and wake up twenty minutes later to answer the pressing question, "I was sweaty an hour ago. Should I go to the hospital?" The only way to survive a whole career is to laugh.

We don't spend our days looking for ways to laugh at our patients. Human beings, however, make it so easy.

Piles of feces dot the carpet. My partner is discreet but inquisitive.

"Sir, do you own a dog?"

"No. Why do you ask?"

My partner waves at the brown piles strewn about like an organic mine field.

The man answers simply, "Oh, yeah. Those are mine."

I bring in a patient who is now combative with Glenn, the nurse assigned to him. As he and two other nurses try to hold the guy down, Glenn looks to me and quips,

"We don't like you anymore. The least you can do is help us restrain him."

I know he is kidding but things will go better for me the next time I bring a patient to this hospital if I do help tie this guy down. I take up the position of lying over the patient's legs with his knees punching me in the abdomen. Glenn leaves to talk to the doctor for an order of Ativan. This guy needs help getting to sleep; he isn't giving up.

Glenn comes back and relates his conversation.

"Can we order up some Ativan for this guy?"

"Yes, give him 0.5 milligrams."

"0.5! Why don't I just go into my bag and give him a breath mint?"

Glenn returns with a bigger order and we are all happy.

Taking care of people is stressful. Patients have their own subtle, individual needs and decisions must be made. This patient needs to be sitting up straight. That patient must stay lying down. The next patient must be strapped to a board and carried down three flights of stairs too narrow to make the turn . . . and he vomits halfway down. Family members swathe their loved one in six layers of clothes while the patient burns with a fever of 103 degrees. I spend half the time pulling clothes off and the family puts them back on because their culture dictates she be covered for warmth. An elderly lady falls, causing a cut to her forehead. She's a little birthday drunk from the celebration of living to ninety. The rules which govern my job say I must strap her ninety-year-old, brittle body to a hard plywood board in case she broke her neck in the fall. She's combative because she thinks the men are coming to take her away. I can only think, *Wonderful, I'm wrestling Grandma.*

Then there's the homeless guy who hates the world and, most especially, anyone wearing a uniform. The reason he's on the street is he took up drinking when his son died thirty years ago. On his sober days he lives in the park, keeps to himself, but doesn't want to follow someone else's rules. When he's drunk — today, next week, and three months from now — he yells at people on "his" street corner. Somebody eventually calls 911. When I step out of the ambulance, both he and his demons legally belong to me. I fight him and them onto the gurney, take him somewhere else, and make the people in the park feel better because they saved this man's life. I take him to the hospital where he punches a nurse before he sobers up, walks out, and starts it all again.

A nurse tries a different tactic with a frequent patient's latest trip to the Emergency Department. A fine, upstanding employee of General Hospital, she brings the patient his food tray. On the tray is a note: "Welcome to Liberty Hospital" — the hospital across town — "We hope you enjoy your meal. Come back and visit us soon."

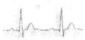

An emergency room patient is in custody and a Sheriff's Deputy is assigned to make sure he stays put.
Patient yelling: "I want two-ply!"
Deputy standing in the hallway yelling back into the room: "Well then, fold it over!"

Whoever said "it takes all kinds of people to make the world go 'round" wasn't kidding.
We are dispatched as an emergency service. We receive the call, speed through traffic while avoiding cars and their inattentive drivers, and use every shortcut permitted by law

to arrive at the address as fast as possible. When asked why they needed an ambulance, some of the responses are:

"I don't have money for a taxi."

"I'm on Medicare so don't worry about your money."

"A very sick man is on my doorstep." In fact, the man turns out to be a homeless person trying to find a place to sleep. The resident calling 911 wants his sidewalk cleared.

We deal with all of humanity. I like it that way. But I think every paramedic and EMT would prefer if the reason we're being sent on a call more often matched up to reality.

Stewart calls 911 so he can hitch a ride to the hospital. He's not sick, he's hungry. He knows how to work the game: Make up a complaint that can't be disproven without a doctor's exam and spin his story enough to at least walk out with a bag lunch.

So the call comes in for his impending seizure. The fire engine and ambulance roll up to find Stewart sitting next to the phone booth two hundred yards from the hospital.

I start off the conversation, "Stewart, what's going on?"

"I'm fixin' to have a seizure."

"Oh, yeah? What makes you think so?"

His answer doesn't matter; this is our normal routine.

But today we have a ride-along, someone interested in the ambulance business and riding with us to learn about it up close. This guy is annoying as hell. He literally steps in between me and my patients during interviews. He desperately wants to fit in and help but he is doing it in the worst way.

Rider Guy stands behind Stewart, part of the circle of firefighters and ambulance folk. He listens to Stewart's tale of woe for the day, reaches out and gently places his hand on Stewart's shoulder. In a quiet and soothing voice he says,

"It's okay. We're just here to help."

Stewart screws his head around, locks in on Rider Guy, and spits out,

"Who the fuck are you?"
My sentiments exactly.

CHAPTER 8

"Wait! I'm Not In Charge!"

College graduation looms and I have a decision to make. This is one of the times in life where I can move anywhere in the world, literally. I already have a job. However, $4.10 an hour isn't going to cut it. California medics are paid $10. I don't realize the price of milk equals the pay difference.

Paramedics and EMTs are governed at the state and county level. They don't exist outside their state lines. To certify in California, I must take a written exam and prove my knowledge. I pass the test allowing me to work in any one of the nine San Francisco Bay Area counties. Heck, I just finished college. I can do a written test. I, however, want a job in Sonoma County and for that I must also take an oral exam: Sit in a room with a doctor and several nurses and get peppered with questions for an hour. Yippee.

I fail the oral—twice. I essentially kill my patient two different times.

This proves I learned the book material but it's not at my fingertips. I had gone through the levels of EMT and paramedic too fast and the belief in what a paramedic can do differs from Alabama to California.

My take on those differences is the attitude about what being a paramedic means. The protocols at the time in Alabama give the impression, "You're just a paramedic, drive them to the hospital and we'll take care of them." The protocols in California seem a bit different. "You're a paramedic. Do what you're trained to do, bring them to the hospital, and we'll continue what you've started." It is a subtle difference but an empowering statement about where I stand in the hierarchy of my patient's care. As for my old stomping grounds? I'm sure things have changed by now.

But now? I'm not going to be a paramedic anymore. I still have a job if I step back and become an EMT... again.

I am no longer starting IVs, no longer administering the medicines, placing the tubes and, more importantly, I am no longer in charge and giving the orders. My job is now as the assistant, tending to my partner's needs. That takes a bit of getting used to.

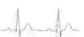

I try to keep the speed down. The firefighters found someone at a fire.

Don't drive too fast. Arriving in one piece is important.

We barrel into town and take a left at the main intersection. The smoke is black and towers to the sky.

We pull into the gravel driveway. I park off to the side in the weeds and throw the gear lever into park. The ambulance has barely stopped moving but Ron and I are both out the doors.

About forty yards in front of us is a mobile home. Well, what is left of one. Orange flames shoot out a window and the black smoke I had followed pours from every seam. Firefighters, dressed in their helmets and coats, hustle back and forth. Some drag hose across the dirt, others shout, wave, and point their needs.

Ron takes off, jumping over swollen fire hose lacing the ground. I run around to the side door of the ambulance to gather the medical box and the oxygen cylinder. These two items take care of most of what we will need.

For what? As a medic I know what I like to take with me on a medical call, but as the EMT, what I want doesn't matter. I am here to support Ron. The one who's not here.

I turn toward the fire.

A firefighter catches my eye. He is running, just like many others, but he seems different. He is running to me. He gets closer and I notice his arms crossed in front of him.

That's a funny way to run. Why is he doing that?

He slows as he comes to me and opens his arms to reveal a baby. "Here, I found her in the trailer."

I look past him. Belching smoke and flames, that trailer is no place from which life should emerge.

I drop my equipment and the firefighter hands me the child. By that action I accepted a patient.

She easily fits into my crossed arms. She is warm. Not cute, cuddly warm. She is toasted warm from being in the trailer and nearly swallowed by flames. Her cheeks are smeared with soot, her eyes closed, and her body is limp.

What am I supposed to do with this? Where's Ron?

I spin in the dirt and gravel hoping to spot him.

I'm supposed to be the partner. I'm just the assistant. Ron's the guy in charge. I'm not a medic anymore. I proved to a whole room of doctors and nurses I wasn't any good at it. Damn! Why was I handed a dead baby?

There is way too much going on. I need the comfort of my ambulance, where everything is laid out perfectly; where I can lay the patient down on a gurney, with sheets. Where I can control the lights and where I can shut the doors to control the noise.

I try not to trip as I step inside and lay the girl down on the gurney. The firefighter who brought her to me stands at the side door of the ambulance. He fills the doorway with his bulky turnouts and helmet. The seconds tick by and it becomes clear I am the one expected to do something.

I drove here in the ambulance. The firefighter found me, the ambulance guy. He doesn't realize, or care, that I'm not the paramedic. I'm not wearing a bright, red beanie blinking in neon, "Not the guy in charge." I am wearing the same uniform as Ron. You know, we all look alike.

I force myself to focus. The ABCs. The letters stand for airway, breathing, and circulation; the basic approach to any patient and the only way I can wrap my mind around this.

I shake the child.

Yep, she's unconscious.

I am supposed to move on to airway and breathing but I wonder if this is a live patient or really a dead child. I slip a finger to the side of her neck.

Hey! There is a pulse!

My mind races. Her little face is smeared with soot as she lies on the gurney. She is wearing a white top with straps over the shoulders. Her mom is going to have to bleach it....

Stop. Keep focused. Her breathing. Is she breathing?

I push her shirt up on her chest. Her belly is not moving up and down. Her chest is not moving.

I need a BVM, a bag-valve-mask. At this level of medical care we, as caregivers, don't do mouth-to-mouth. We don't need to; we use the equipment for that. The bag-valve-mask is all the name implies. I squeeze the bag to force oxygen through the valve and into the mask over the patient's face. My patient isn't breathing. I must do it for her.

The BVM is in a cabinet on the other end of the ambulance. My next action is clear, but I struggle with a problem.

I should get the BVM.

She hasn't been breathing for a while. She needs air now.

I hate doing mouth to mouth!

The firefighter doesn't know where it's kept. That leaves me.

I don't want to leave my patient.

I mentally bounce back and forth across the ambulance getting the BVM and not getting the BVM.

Make a decision!

More firefighters crowd at the back door of the ambulance. They are in a better position for what I need.

I yell out to no one in particular.

"I need a BVM! Somebody grab me a BVM!"

I keep shaking the girl, trying to stimulate her to breathe. Nothing is happening. I'm also not being handed what I need and she is still not breathing. Life is edging away and I must commit and make a change.

Damn it. Fine. I'm doing mouth-to-mouth.

I had been down this road only four years ago. Doing mouth-to-mouth breathing that time on a dead motorcycle guy, I had been naïve and not done a full exam. This time I realize exactly what I am getting into and why. This girl is not breathing. She is not dead, not yet anyway, but I had better do something.

This is a child about eighteen months old. On adults one is supposed to pinch the nose closed and blow into the mouth. On kids of this size there isn't that much space for all those fingers and lips.

I open my mouth wide and cover her mouth and nose. I shift my head a little until I gain a seal, then I blow air into her lungs. Her chest rises. I feel the resistance of her full lungs and I stop. I blow again and her chest rises with my air into her body. Her skin is soft on my lips. My mouth again seals to her face as I pass my air over. The flavor of soot and the odor of smoke fill my nose. The moisture of my breath causes my lips to lift the grit off her face carried from the fire.

And then Ron is beside me. He lays another child down on the bench and begins to work on him. We have two critical patients. Plenty of firefighters crowd the doors ready to help but there is only so much space to work.

My patient needs to be intubated. She needs a tube to protect her airway from swelling closed after being exposed to the hot gasses of the fire and in case she vomits. Ron is a paramedic. I used to be a medic, but now I'm an EMT. I know how to intubate but I can't do it in this state. If I intubate her and anything goes wrong, I can lose my job, I can lose my EMT certification, and I can lose any chance of becoming a paramedic again. Ron can also lose his certification for letting me do it.

Bending down I give her another breath. Her chest rises and falls in a smooth motion. I'm not going to keep doing mouth-to-mouth on this girl. While it works, a BVM gives me a chance to give her 100% oxygen through the mask.

Besides, tasting the fire and feeling the gritty soot on her soft cheek is just a little too grimy and personal.

I stand, move three steps to the back of the ambulance, slide open a cabinet and grab a pediatric bag-valve-mask. The bag and the mask are smaller and made for children. My hands shake while I assemble the parts. My patient is not breathing while I put the bag together.

Done. I plug the tubing into the wall port and spin the dial up to fifteen liters per minute. With the mask over her face, my thumb and forefinger around the mask, I hold on to her jaw with the rest of my fingers. Air escapes from around her lips each time I squeeze the bag. A little adjustment and her cheeks fill the space under the soft ring of the mask. My job now is to breathe for her once every three seconds.

My mind moves and forms a list of needs for the girl.

She's got a pulse and I'm breathing for her. She's still unconscious which means she still needs to be intubated. However, I can't do that for her. The BVM will have to do for now. She also needs an IV. If her heart fails, she will need drugs to bring her back. I can't do that, either.

Damn, this is frustrating! The whole list of things to do hovers in front of me and I can't do any of it.

I'm usually a patient and mellow guy. But, when something slows down the care for my patient, I get pissed. Now the speed bump is me.

Ron is busy with his own patient. This isn't the time to burden him with my issues. He slips the laryngoscope blade into the boy's mouth. I've done many intubations. I'm actually pretty good at them. When Ron lifts the jaw I can visualize his view of the patient's vocal cords. He must be careful not to rock the handle back. He could break the boy's teeth. A firm but gentle upward pull is needed and the throat opens up.

Once Ron sees the inverted "V" of the vocal cords, he inserts the tube into the tiny mouth, never taking his eyes off the cords, and passes the tube between the arms of the "V."

Ron finishes tying the tube down on his patient and begins pressing oxygen in using another BVM. He glances over at me and says,

"Whatchya got over there?"

"A firefighter brought her over to me while you were gone looking for your patient. She is unresponsive but has a pulse. I couldn't find a Pedi-BVM in time so I had to do mouth-to-mouth on her."

I squeeze the bag every few seconds to keep my patient oxygenated while I sample the soot and grime I will revisit over the next week.

Ron examines the limp girl on the gurney.

"It looks like she's stabilized now. She could still use a tube. Here, switch with me."

We trade places. Ron waves a firefighter into the ambulance.

"I need you to bag her while I get my stuff ready to intubate."

The firefighter kneels down on the end of the gurney to take the bag from Ron. She is so small. Ron and the firefighter almost touch heads as they work. Ron assembles his equipment for another intubation while I bag my new patient.

The BVM is easy to squeeze and the boy's chest rises and falls each time. He must be an older brother. He is about five. His clothes are still on, an orange t-shirt with blue jeans. His face and arms are smudged with soot. At least he isn't burned by the fire like the girl. It appears the smoke and hot gas got him.

Ron drops the tube into the throat of the girl and tapes it down. The firefighter takes the face mask off the BVM and puts the bag's connector directly on the tube snaking into her throat.

Ron continues to direct his chaotic scene. First, he speaks to the firefighter bagging the infant.

"You switch with me and sit here. Do you mind if we borrow you to go to the hospital? We'll bring you back."

The firefighter shakes his head.

"Sure. It looks like your hands are full."

"Thank you."

Ron asks the group gathered outside the door of the ambulance.

"I need one more helper, please."

Another firefighter hops in.

Ron directs him over to me as he says,

"If you can take over bagging that patient, we'll get going to the hospital."

He turns to me as I step out the side door.

"Okay, Scott. Let's go."

I climb back into the driver's seat and we rocket off to the hospital. Ron starts an IV on both patients while I try to keep the ambulance smooth but swift. If I can't do anything else, at least I can try to keep the bumps out. I fight the urge to drive faster.

At the hospital we turn our patients over to the waiting nurses and doctor. We leave after cleaning up and doing paperwork, then take the firefighters back to their station. The patients? I don't know if they live.

That evening Ron and I go out for dinner at the local pizza joint. I am halfway through when the shakes start. The horror is finally coming to the surface. I did mouth-to-mouth on a child. You only do mouth-to-mouth, for real, on people who are almost dead. I can still smell the fire and smoke. I can still taste her. I tasted death.

I'm also struggling with what I couldn't do for the little girl. I used to be a paramedic. I used to be able to put my ambulance to its full use. The tools are there and I, at one time, could pull magic out of a hat to save a life.

Now, I can see what needs to be done and I must sit on my hands and wait for my partner. Ron's a good medic, I'm right there with him. But, today, my girl could have gotten better. I failed and I don't even know if she lived through what I couldn't give her.

Ron calls our local counselor for emergency workers and I go through my first debriefing. It saves my life.

One and a half years later I find out the baby girl lived, the one I did mouth-to-mouth on. She lost some toes but she is alive. Fifteen years later, through a sheer coincidence, I find out her brother also lived. I meet her again and she's a wonderful teenage girl.

CHAPTER 9

"Yeah, But The View!"

How I met my wife, Camille. She was a nurse at one of the emergency departments, cute and single. I asked her out on a date and she said, "Maybe."

I didn't give up. Eventually, she couldn't resist, and a few years later I asked her to marry me. She said yes.

In addition to falling in love, I was going to paramedic school—again. I had been an EMT for four years and the time had come to get back on the horse. I was lucky enough to do my training in San Francisco for the Department of Public Health, Paramedic Division, which offered great experiences for a student. Things happened in big cities that didn't seem to happen anywhere else.

I was assigned to work on unit 92-A with Matt and Jason. They were serious and got the job done when needed, but we laughed a lot between times. We started our shift at three-thirty in the afternoon by checking out the ambulance and restocking items from the morning shift. Twenty minutes later we were given an area of the city to cover and expected to run calls until finished at one-thirty in the morning. We didn't get the easy calls. We got whatever came out of the radio with our number.

Today's assignment was Union Square. Jason wandered somewhere among the food stands and street hawkers while Matt and I dug into my textbooks, discussing the finer points of congestive heart failure.

"Ninety-two Adam. Got one for ya."

Richard was in Dispatch. His monotone voice, no inflection, no excitement, dropped out of the speaker. Some people believed he stayed up nights perfecting his delivery.

Matt answered back with our unit ID and location in a purposefully chipper voice.

"Ninety-two Adam! The Square!"

It didn't work on Richard.

"Ninety-two Adam. Code 2 for the eight-oh-two, number one Sutter, apartment ten-oh-two on one-six-seven."

Matt tried again, this time with a little levity.

"Copy. *Number* one Sutter, *number* ten-oh-two on *number* one-six-seven. En route."

Richard was done with us.

"Ninety-two Adam, en route. Break. Ninety-five, copy Code 3."

When I first started my training I asked Matt and Jason about the codes and numbers they used. Each city I worked in so far used its own police, fire, and medical codes. Also, the paperwork and tracking info was unique to each department and employer. While learning how to be a medic again I was also expected to learn the special language of San Francisco.

The number 167 was actually the last three digits of a six-digit number started five years before. At the beginning of the shift we put the full number on the log sheet but, for the rest of the day, Dispatch and the log only reflected the last three numbers, growing one by one, as they were assigned to each call system-wide.

802 was cop talk for a dead body. For 100 years the ambulance service in San Francisco has been tossed from one parent department to another. At one time the paramedics used to be under the umbrella of the police and we still used a few of their codes to keep the scanner hounds from knowing about our response to a dead body. We also used 800 for a psychiatrically unstable person and 801 for a suicide attempt.

Matt put the microphone back in its cradle. He turned the portable radio clipped on his belt to another channel, one that didn't repeat over the entire city.

"Hey, Jason. We've got an eight-oh-two on Sutter."

I closed my books and readied myself for the drive to Sutter Street. When Jason returned we could be there in about three minutes.

Matt grabbed his cooler and left the ambulance. One of the nearby food stands either liked us or took pity and let us use their microwave to heat up our meals. That left me alone, waiting to drive toward our pending call.

I looked around my domain, at the gurney and the cabinets filled with the tools of medicine I was supposed to master. Richard's monotone voice droned from the radio in the cab. With ours off his monitor we no longer mattered as the minutes ticked by and we didn't move. We hadn't turned the key or even come together as a full crew while someone waited for us to show up at their door, our bags in hand, ready to solve their problem. When Matt got back I asked him my pressing questions.

"Matt, an eight-oh-two is a dead body call, right?"

"Yeah."

"First, why are we even going? Second, if we are going, why aren't we moving a little faster in case somebody messed up and the guy's not really dead?"

Matt answered between his bites of chicken and pasta. His wife was a good cook, from the smell. My cooler held a sandwich.

"The City and County of San Francisco have decided to sort of make us Deputy Coroners. They need help processing dead bodies. We start the process and then call them. True, somebody may not be able to recognize dead when they see it. But, we have to go with the information we've been given and respond appropriately. If we didn't, we'd be zipping all over town going Code 3 for every little inane complaint because we've decided we can't trust any information. That's not safe for us or the public, having us drive fast and busting red lights when we don't need to.

"So, this is a Code 2 call, this guy's not getting any deader and, according to the Paramedic Division's rules, we've got twenty minutes to arrive on scene. Sutter Street is right around the corner, Jason's not back yet from his shopping, and I'm hungry. Might as well eat while I can."

I guess so.

Jason returned with a diminishing coffee. Matt buckled himself in and then washed his hands using the alcohol towelettes provided by the Division to cleanse between calls.

At about ten o'clock on a gorgeous spring evening, we drove slowly over to the end of Sutter Street and climbed out. Jason knocked on the glass door of the lobby. The doorman buzzed us in with a practiced flourish, directed us to the waiting elevator, and left us with a final direction.

"Ten-oh-two will be on your right as you exit."

The doors shut and we began the trip while Jason made a big show of sitting on the very plush couch placed in the corner of our little rising room. I set the jump kit and heart monitor on the hardwood floor. Matt held the clipboard.

I only brought the jump kit because I always brought the jump kit. This person was dead. We were just going for paperwork but I hated surprises. I might be a student with Matt and Jason, however I've already been doing this job long enough to know surprises might mean mouth-to-mouth and I'm not doing that on anybody again.

I brought the heart monitor for a few reasons. First, I was being evaluated and must show I was thinking of all angles and possibilities. The remote possibility was this guy wasn't truly dead and somebody had missed that fact. The more reasonable possibility had our patient not showing enough signs of obvious death, like rigor mortis, or displaced important parts, and I needed to patch him up and show a straight-line strip to the medical examiner guys.

The elevator doors opened and we took the suggested right turn to enter the second of only two apartments on the floor. The thick carpet and walls covered in paintings and mirrors joined the wallpaper in perfectly appointed harmony. The furniture gleamed and everything sparkled.

Opulence costs money and in this home I couldn't afford a spoon.

The police, already spaced about the apartment and interviewing the boyfriend, pointed me to the bedroom. I followed the indicated direction and stepped inside the room to find more money well-spent. Glass and a floral pattern dominated the theme and I hugged my street-worn bags a little closer.

I rounded the bed to do my exam and dropped my equipment to the carpet. The lower they were, the safer. The thud of bags to floor was barely heard.

The dead lady, looking somewhere in her fifties, lay on her right side on top of the comforter as she sank into her last resting place of a chartreuse sateen floral pattern. Her eyes had the blank and glossed look I was beginning to recognize too often, and her face wore the stillness of sleeping without the color of life.

I began my search for signs of death with her eyelids. Yes, they felt stiff. Rigor mortis begins in the small muscles. I moved on to her fingers. Stiff as well. I lifted her shirt and leaned over to view her back. A subtle, but perceptible tinge of blue rose up a few inches on her lower side. Lividity is the pooling of the blood no longer pushed around the body by the heart. It settles to the lowest point. For the completeness of the medical examiner's report I patched her up with the three leads and ran a strip of what I fully expected, asystole.

I stepped back to make a further assessment and guess the cause of her death. The vomit on her shirt crafted a blood-colored tinge and matched the large quantity of vomit/blood sprayed over the corner of the room.

A thorough search of the apartment would be disturbing the scene but I lay odds I could find many empty bottles of vodka. Over the years, her drinking had eaten her intestines from the inside out until she bled to death internally. Her final moments had been a violent rejection of that lifestyle. The police in the next room were only needed to preserve the evidence for the medical examiner; they would not be taking the boyfriend away in dramatic TV crime drama fashion.

I, being the student, got to do the paperwork. I just needed to hear the story from the cops and the boyfriend about what had happened, when he had last seen her alive, and were there any medical complaints. I wrote it all down for the medical examiner guys who would be arriving soon.

When finished I walked into the living room. Matt and Jason stood in front of the plate glass window stretching the entire length of the room. Before us lay the most incredible view.

San Francisco is a beautiful city. The view equals the amount of money you can spend and this lady had spent a lot. It began on the left side with the Golden Gate Bridge. Below us, the lights from the waterfront of San Francisco sparkled while the cities of Richmond and Berkeley across the bay filled the middle. The San Francisco/Oakland Bay Bridge bounded the right side. It was stunning.

Then the boyfriend started sobbing behind us and didn't stop. The volume of his grief spread throughout the room. I glanced to my right and took note that Matt and Jason appeared unfazed by the wailing behind us. When did that happen in the career of a paramedic?

We had been dispatched here to make official the death of a lady. We had done that. Our work was finished and I, as the student, executed my duties well for tonight's performance review. But this was a learning moment, also. I looked to Matt and Jason to learn how an experienced medic took on the extra duty of helping a grieving family member. So far they didn't appear to care.

My stomach churned with every fresh sob and I played out different solutions in my head. We carried nothing in our equipment that would solve this problem. This man did not need our services of transport to an emergency room. What were we expected to do? Were we expected to do anything?

In the room gathered just the cops, us, and the boyfriend. The officers kept looking at the guy, then glancing our way. Finally, Matt and Jason dispatched me to tend to him. I went over with my jump kit and knelt to meet him as he lay curled on the floor. Maybe some medical procedures like taking his blood pressure would help as I did my best to console him through the fresh moments of his loss.

"Yes, sir, I know you love her."

"But, the pain . . . I'm going to miss her so much." He hugged himself tight to contain the turmoil.

"Yes, it does hurt. The pain will lessen slightly with each day but hold on to those memories. They're precious."

"But I love her." He sobbed into the carpet.

"Yes, sir. And you still can. Remember the joy and fun."

With no success over several minutes, Matt came over and I let him slide into the caregiver role.

I went back with Jason, tried to tune out the boyfriend, and gave thought to this whole scene.

It is the job of a paramedic to wade into the lives and emergencies of others. The anguish thrown off from these events is real and if I became emotionally involved in every heartbreaking moment, every tit for tat argument, all the tales that take the normal person down to becoming a destitute drug-ridden food scrabbler living on the sidewalk, I wouldn't last. Sure, I could strain to help the few I come across in their myriad and complex needs before I burnt out, but I wanted to be a paramedic for a long time. To do that I had to realize what I can do and what I can offer.

I carried a bag filled with equipment and medicine. These tools were not everything a doctor could do for his patient but with my training I could do more with those tools than the banker guy walking down the street. The same goes for my toolbox of emotional support. I couldn't offer everything a psychiatrist could, but I did have the skills to offer a little and to know when I was done.

I stood next to Jason, mulled these thoughts over, listened to Matt in his attempts to calm the boyfriend, and took in the absolutely stunning view. I could see for miles. The twinkling lights of Oakland sparkled like jewels off the water of the bay. The lighthouse on Alcatraz Island scribed a circle and flashed when it crossed our plane. The continuous stream of headlights coming across the Bay Bridge formed a moving line strung below the graceful necklace of lights sweeping from each tower. Matt came back to our side. The boyfriend still wailed and it was Jason's turn.

The other side of this coin, the life of a medic as we triaged our way through the emotions and needs of our patients, was to realize the glory of life in front of us. One must acknowledge the wonder of newborn life even as it emerges from a rain-soaked sidewalk gutter. The rush of efficiency must receive a hat-tip when the hospital stops the bleeding and saves the life of the man you brought them who had been deeply stabbed.

Here too, Jason, Matt, and I must stop and pay heed to the beauty of the view before us while offering what we could to soften the fresh grief in this man's life. It was all a balancing act and what we do as paramedics. I tuned out the boyfriend as Jason did his work.

The fog coming in through the Golden Gate snuck in just above the water line and below the bridge. The main bank hung just offshore, ready to pounce and envelop the bridge in its entirety. The tall buildings of downtown stood in the foreground around us. The lights of those still at work in each building set a mosaic checkerboard to the streets far below. What a view.

CHAPTER 10

The Cardiac

After training in San Francisco, I received my paramedic license and went back to Santa Rosa. I got my old job, not as an EMT but as a medic, worked for two years, and started taking on students as a paramedic instructor. During a student's one-year program, he or she is scrutinized by all levels of healthcare professionals; the last two to four months are with me on my ambulance. I give them an environment to practice making choices and trying out different ideas about how to work with people in their worst moments. I also create a place where they can make mistakes and I will catch them before any harm comes to the patient. As the instructor, I enjoy watching the blossoming of a new medic while I stand across the room making sure everything is done correctly, despite the student's lack of experience. Tom, my latest young sprout, was almost finished.

I drove the ambulance through the weeds and over crunching gravel, trying to stay off the railroad ties. Beating the axle to death over the rotting lumber wouldn't be good. Dispatch said we'd find our patient next to the tracks complaining of chest pain: A cardiac. We could have parked at the road, grabbed our equipment and walked in until we found him. But it was late in the week, getting late in the day, and driving seemed a good idea at the time.

I picked my way along, adjusting to avoid pockets of deeper gravel, until a woman stepped out of the high grass ahead of us. Her tall, thin frame, bulked up by several layers of clothing, was topped off by a long, black, ratty coat that lay open to the warm autumn day. Dark hair, mimicking her coat, hung past her thin face. Barely out of

83

the grass, she cocked a stance bigger than her clothes, sucked on a cigarette, and seemed to smolder the phrase, *Fuck this shit.*

I rolled up next to her and shut down the engine. Dave, my partner, and Tom popped out to meet our reporting party as I crawled out the driver's side. The fire engine crew walked down the tracks to join us while Tom and Dave followed the lady and disappeared into the weeds. I rounded the back of the ambulance and did the same until a massive figure being led, sort of, came toward me.

Our patient, I gathered, stumbled from the bushes with Dave and Tom flanking him, each clinging to an arm. Their attempts to lead the man were valiant. But truthfully, they were just light weights hanging off a side of beef, occasionally jostling it back to the center of its trajectory. In a few more steps, like the giant from *Jack and the Beanstalk*, the man's feet entangled and his upper body pitched forward, suggesting an imminent crash. I reached out and grabbed a hunk of pant leg to assist. Not a good idea.

The guy was a man's man; a rock able to navigate life without any help. Of course his current level of navigating provided an enchanting ground floor view of the weeds next to defunct railroad tracks but, hey, he was a man of his own destiny.

"Fuck off," he said, as he kicked at me.

My continued presence only caused problems and Tom was far enough in his training he needed the experience of handling tough patients. I backed off, sat on the bumper of the ambulance, chatted with the fire crew and kept an eye out while Tom and Dave struggled to jostle the man inside.

Then a call came in for a car fire across the street. I took stock. Things still flowed toward the ambulance.

I said to the firefighters, "You guys go. Have fun."

They were off.

Tom and Dave got our guy inside and I weighed my role in this. The patient and I were not getting along. Tom, despite his inexperience, was doing pretty well, and since Dave is a paramedic, the decision was clear.

I announced, "Hey guys, I'm driving on this one." I shut the back door.

I directed the lady to hop in the front with me. She tossed her cigarette to the tracks and climbed in the passenger seat.

I pulled myself in using the steering wheel and said, "Could you put on your seat belt, please?"

She secured the buckle across her chest, turned sideways, and yelled to the back, "I'm right here, honey. I'm with you."

"He's getting the best care available. He'll be fine."

She didn't relax and she didn't turn around. They never do. Okay, off to the hospital.

I dropped the gear shift into drive and slowly picked my way along the tracks even while the gravel got thick. I went faster, trying to float a little, until the ambulance started to fishtail and sink. I grew up in Ohio and driving in the snow was worse than this. Only a few yards to go . . . until the rear descended into the gravel.

Damn. I almost made it. Time to reassess.

Should I call the supervisor? No, not yet. There was still a chance to escape from this unscathed. The planning ended when a voice suggesting a restrained, but vicious, dog wafted from the back.

"Let me out now or I kick the door open."

Everybody out.

I stepped out and surveyed the depth of the problem. We sat buried to the axle. The patient appeared at the back of the ambulance. His long hair hung in his face while his eyes, which before were rheumy and unfocused, now shone bright and pissed off. I faced a bear I awoke from hibernation.

He took a square stance, pointed right at me and growled, "You. Come over here. I've got something I want to say to you."

Through concealed panic I yelled back, "If you've got something to say, you can say it from there."

He weaved and wiped the hair from his face. I held rock still, trying not to pee my pants. Over the next few seconds his thoughts and steam lost momentum, then his eyes chose another plan and he barked out an order, "Just get in the front."

I liked that idea. *What did I do to piss this guy off?*

I climbed in, slammed the door, and locked the ambulance. I locked Dave and Tom outside with him but that didn't seem to be a problem for them.

The side mirror displayed our cardiac patient who, until a few moments ago appearing too drunk to walk, helped to dig out the ambulance. Also, an army of homeless folk descended upon us to make this a community project. Much yelling and directing filled the air. Wood became re-appropriated from a business next door to be stuffed under the tires. Our patient shifted gravel and worked quite hard until he ran forward to yell at me through the window, unshaven, hair dangling in unwashed strands over his eyes, and still enormous.

"When I tell you to, hit it."

That sounded like a plan.

From outside and near the back I heard, "Okay, hit it."

So I did. Gravel shot everywhere.

The shouts from behind were clear.

"Fuck! Damn it! Shit!"

He ran back to my window and continued yelling.

"Stop. Stop!"

I checked my exit out the other door. I would have to climb over the console and a computer. In a pinch, no issue. I heard another barrage of orders.

"Hit it."

So I did.

"Fuck, damn, shit! Stop. Stop!"

I stopped.

The fire engine crew, finished battling their car blaze, saw our trouble and came back. They brought tools. Through the mirror I noted the shovels and rakes stayed in fire department hands and I prayed a thank you. Tools can be weapons. Mr. Large and I still didn't have closure. Oh, and the supervisor had found us. He stood, his massive arms folded over his chest, next to Dave, and they were talking between themselves. This was not going well.

"Okay, hit it."

This time I rose out of the gravel, drove to the cross street and back on the road which paralleled the railroad tracks, the one where we should have parked before.

As far as I was concerned, we were free and clear. This man could do whatever he wanted and go wherever he pleased. I could write a patient care report to cover us. I wasn't to be the one convincing him of anything. Our patient, however, had taken a liking to one of the fire engine crew members and she talked him into going to the hospital.

Dave told me later about his side of the whole debacle.

I was hunkered inside the ambulance for safety. Dave called the supervisor, then stood at a safe distance while the digging progressed with our patient giving the orders. The supervisor arrived, and Tom, still believing he controlled the call, approached to present a briefing on the situation. Brushing past the intern like a charging rhino in size and style, the supe headed toward the ambulance and the melee surrounding it. He noticed Dave, redirected, stopped when he reached Dave's vantage point, faced the action, and then crossed his arms over his beefy chest.

Dave said, his arms also crossed over his chest, "Hey, Boss."

The supervisor responded, not joyfully, "What in the hell is going on?"

"Well, you see that behemoth pushing with exuberance on the ambulance?"

"Yes." Still not cheerily.

"That is our patient and he is complaining of chest pain which, as you know, should not be made worse with exercise. My plan is to get the ambulance unstuck and then ask him, politely, to get back inside. He will refuse.

"I will then call the Base Hospital to do a patient refusal. The doctor will tell me because the patient is complaining of chest pain he must go. I will relay the message and the patient will tell me to go to hell.

"The doctor will tell me to get him to sign a refusal form. The patient will refuse to sign the form, quite possibly threatening me, and I will tell the doctor this. I will request someone else sign as a witness, thank the doctor for his time, all paperwork will be finished, and we will go away."

The supervisor was happy. About then I rose from the depths of our problem, drove around the block, and the firefighter sweet-talked the man into going to the hospital.

Damn it!

Fine. We all got in. This time, however, we made a few shifts in seating. We moved the girlfriend to the back to keep our patient happy. We added the man's new friend, the firefighter, back there, along with Dave, to keep things official. Besides, Dave hadn't pissed anybody off. Yet.

I had lost all control of the call and Tom sat up front with me where we discussed how to dodge the multitude of legal storms possible to arise from this incident through artful, but factually correct, wording on the patient care report. For instance, we would only mention that the patient's chest pain did not worsen with exercise which, most often, is measured against a simple task, like walking across the room. Not, shall we say, working up a sweat while digging the ambulance out of the gravel it may have been stuck in.

I congratulated Tom on his attempts to keep the call rolling and trying to brief the supervisor. We also reviewed safety procedures and the fact we are number one on that list. We are not trained, nor can we be expected, to take unnecessary risks to subdue a patient and convince him to follow our plan of action. There comes a point, I had showcased very well myself, when we step out of the way. We finished and delivered the patient to the nurses.

The fire engine crew, the supervisor, Dave, Tom, and I chatted outside the emergency room when the patient came barreling out the doors. He burst through us all and stormed off to the street with his girlfriend skittering behind. I hadn't even finished the patient care report for the hospital. Also, while I didn't look forward to it, I was sure I had an incident report to do after this.

I turned in the paperwork to the nurse's station and stepped outside to receive my reprimand and assignment to have an incident report on his desk by the end of shift. Instead, the supervisor gave me a look, something along the lines of, "That won't be happening again, will it?"

He was a temporary supervisor that day. He didn't want to do the paperwork, either.

CHAPTER 11

James Richards

We picked up James sometimes twice in a week or even twice in a day. I cracked jokes about our frequent fliers by saying if they get enough mileage points they win a toaster.

Some helpful citizen called us to save him and we'd find him lying with his feet stuck out from behind a bush. Honestly? People wanted to be rid of him. He cluttered up their bush.

I'd get out of the ambulance and give James a nudge. "Hey. Wake up."

Probably in his thirties — hard to tell — James was lanky and tall with scraggly blonde hair. If he was sober enough, we sat him up and found out his needs, offered a trip to the hospital, and gave him a blanket on cold mornings. Some days he didn't smell bad. Other days, after pulling a heavy drunk and not having a bath recently, he could stink up some serious acreage.

My job was to check and make sure he hadn't hurt himself. I would examine his head to see if he fell, pull up his shirt looking for signs of being assaulted, catalog for this time, and the next, his list of bruises and cuts.

James was a drunk.

We labeled our calls, it's easier: The cardiac; the SOB (shortness of breath); the psych. We viewed only a piece, in some it was the rubble, of our patients' lives. The malady or situation for which we were called consumed the debris we attempted to right. "Drunk," however, became a persona.

Of course James wasn't always a drunk. He once owned a little red wagon. His blond hair would have swung lightly in the breeze and maybe he pulled it back in a ponytail as he kissed a girlfriend. At some point James developed a drinking problem which consumed his life.

We extracted James from behind the bush and loaded him into the ambulance. We did a cursory physical exam to check for other reasons to be unconscious, like being shot or stabbed, took vital signs, and checked his blood sugar to prove diabetes was not the reason for his unconsciousness. We rolled him on his side in case he threw up and let him sleep on the way to the hospital.

In the emergency department I turned James over to the nurse and stepped off to do paperwork while the doctor decided to either let him sleep it off or direct the nurse to start an IV and give him a "banana bag." The banana bag was a collection of liquid vitamins that, when mixed, took on the yellow hue of a banana. Alcoholism is very hard on the body, sapping a lot of nutrients; then there's the poor diet.

The nurse attempted to start an IV, usually done in an arm vein. They are the least painful and easiest. She tried to find a vein in one arm, then the other. Carol was a solid nurse. The patient had no IV if she couldn't get one. James lay splayed on the gurney as she took a few stabs, gave up, and moved to his feet. While a viable alternative, foot veins hurt a lot more to put in, rousing James from his stupor.

Some people are vocal about their pain and choose a colorful vocabulary and I expected this from James.

Half-risen in the bed, he loudly stated to the nurse with each jab, "Thank you! Thank you!"

Three weeks later James lay in the bed of another hospital, one of many where he spent time. I transported a patient in and spied him sitting up, appearing sober.

Finished with my patient and the paperwork, I walked into James' room. I didn't know if he knew me or my face. I may have just been a guy wearing a uniform, one that showed up often in his life.

"Good afternoon, James."

"Good afternoon."

"How are you feeling today?"

"Aw, alright, I guess."

"I took you into Memorial a few weeks ago and you acted in a way that caught me by surprise. I thought I would share with you."

I related the story to him about his words to the nurse and how I was amazed he chose not to cuss his way through the ordeal.

He answered, "Well, yeah. I may be a drunk but I'm not an asshole."

James' life ended one chilly morning on a park bench. A friend of mine pronounced him dead.

I wish I would have gotten that call.

CHAPTER 12

Daryl Robert Preston

I walk fast toward my patient. Tended by the knot of firefighters around him, he lay on the crest of the street, stripped to his underwear, and on the backboard. With a shooting, I want to be done and out in less than ten minutes. Thanks to the fire engine crew, today we'd be done in five.

A well-run trauma call is efficient, creating speed. When one flows exactly right, I absorb the entire patient at once while my hands search and find miniscule details. I hear the tiniest aberration in the patient's lungs. I perceive all movements of the crew, before they're made. I am a robot. I am faster than is possible. I can see the future and that feels amazing. Like cocaine to an addict.

I straddle the patient and begin my physical exam before we all find ourselves stuffed into the back of the ambulance and before things get busy.

Hair and facial area, clear. Left ear, through-and-through wound. Nothing to worry about. Eyes, open. He's gasping for air.

He sputters, "I can't breathe. I can't breathe, man."

I translate his words into his medical condition. *He's breathing. He's talking. Good brain function.*

I give him an answer to let him know I'm listening.

"We're going to take care of you. Hold on."

Keep moving. Don't slow down.

A brief check of the neck. *Nothing spectacular.* I move my hands away and a firefighter follows with a cervical collar.

Arms. *Grazing shot, left upper arm. Nothing on the left lower.* Move to the right arm. *There's one. Right upper.* Check the armpits. *Got one. Right chest, under the arm.*

The adrenalin courses through me.

God, I love it when I catch the tough ones.

I admonish myself. *Move! Work!*

Right lower arm. *Nothing.* To the hands.

I place two fingers in each of the man's palms and tell him firmly, "Squeeze." He grabs them, hard. I shake him loose, continuing my search at the chest.

Keep slow. Check everything. Bullet holes are small.

My gloved hands touch every bit of his skin, even purposely sloshing through puddles of blood on his chest.

Found one. Off-center to the right.

I continue on and, like a macabre finger painting, I leave bloody swirls down to his stomach.

I push on the four abdominal quadrants. My hands press deep without a problem. *Belly is clear.* I rock his hips back and forth while pressing down, then in. *Pelvis intact.*

I shift his underwear around, trying to maintain a shred of modesty for this guy, but I pore over every inch of his body in the expanse of the intersection. *One hole in the left butt.* Shift on down. *Another one, left thigh.*

I finish my assessment by yelling, "Move your feet."

His toes wriggle. Responds to commands.

I stand and my back burns as the strain subsides.

The fire guys strap him to the backboard while I strip off my bloody gloves and drop them between his legs. I'll put on new ones in the ambulance.

Damn, this guy's got...one,,, two... three... My fingers follow the progression of bullet holes I have found... *four... five.,. six... seven holes in him. Who'd he piss off?*

I never did examine his back. He needs a surgeon more than me rolling him off the board. Besides, he's shutting off any holes back there by lying on them. My partner rolls the gurney beside us. Time to go.

"Okay, everybody, on three."

Four uniforms snap to their places around the board.

"One, two, three."

Our patient sails up and onto the gurney. The straps fairly fly to buckle him down. We roll to the ambulance.

I jump inside.

Keep things flowing. We're moving steady. Only do important things; skip the fluff.

One of the firefighters, Ron, jumps in the back with me. He sits behind the patient's head and I start barking orders as I put on fresh gloves.

"High flow oxygen by mask. I've got the heart monitor."

Ron rips open a cabinet and grabs a non-rebreather mask. I shift to grab the heart monitor but stop. I haven't listened to this guy's lungs yet and it's about to get a lot noisier in here when we start driving.

I place the stethoscope in my ears and lean over the patient, bracing myself on the opposite wall.

I sternly call out, "Take a deep breath. In and out."

Our man's chest rises up and down.

"A couple more."

I move the scope over his chest, hearing full and equal breath sounds on both sides.

"Thank you."

Some of those bullets definitely hit lung tissue. I'm pleased either the important stuff was missed or he hasn't degraded enough to show it. Ron drops the mask over our patient's face and adds a strip of tape securing a seal.

"I can't breathe. I can't breathe."

The mask muffles the guy's protests.

I try to calm him a little as I toss the stethoscope back in the bag.

"That is oxygen, man. Pure oxygen. Leave the mask on. Keep breathing."

Don't let him distract you. Be efficient. That's his best chance.

I reach over to the heart monitor and pull the cords from the pouch, the three patches hooked on already. I rip them off in order, slap them on his chest, and flip the dial on the machine. The green blip flows across the screen, giving a constant reading of his heart rate at 136. That is fast but he now sports seven new holes.

I yell out to my partner, "Time to go. Drive smooth! We're working back here."

My next duties are to call the hospital and start an IV. With enough time, I might even try a blood pressure. As long as he has a pulse at his wrist I honestly don't care. His pressure's high enough.

However, an IV, with all the packaging, tubing connections and sterile technique, takes time to set up. Once done, I have to find a vein, clean the site, stick the needle into the vein in a moving vehicle and hook up the IV. That usually takes me about five minutes. I have four.

I look up. Bill, my partner, flooded an IV while we packaged this guy. The bag and tubing hang from the hook above my head. I love working with a good partner.

I yell to the front of the ambulance, "Hey, Bill. Can you call the hospital? We've got a lot to do back here."

Bill yells back, "Sure. You've got about three minutes."

I shift down to prep our patient's left arm for the IV. I rip and tear packages, lay the contents out then stretch the tourniquet around his upper arm and tie it snug.

"I can't breathe. I just can't breathe."

I glance at the man's chest. He's breathing way too fast. His skin is now pale and he is sweating.

Damn, he's getting worse.

"Ron, can you grab the BVM? He needs to be bagged."

Ron reaches into the jump kit on the floor and pulls out the bag-valve-mask. He yanks the non-rebreather off the patient, throwing it aside and then places the BVM's mask over the guy's face. Ron squeezes the bag and forces 100 percent oxygen into the man's lungs.

I search for a vein. This guy is young, he seems about thirty, but his body type is one with a fine layer of fat all over. Enough to hide his veins.

"I can't breathe, man."

Ahh, not again, I yell to myself in frustration.

I look up. The guy's eyes bulge with fright; his mouth gasps for air. He rocks back and forth against the belts holding him.

Something isn't right. This guy's breathing problems are slowing me down. The basic approach to medicine at any level is called the ABCs, a mnemonic for Airway, Breathing, and Circulation. If I don't solve one, don't move on to the next. Solving "B" stubbornly fixes itself as my main issue ever since we got into the ambulance. I keep looking for a vein while, in my head, I run through the problem like two guys screaming at each other.

His lungs are clear. The air is getting to the lungs. Why can't he breathe?

He took two bullets to the chest. His lungs are hit.

But I heard air all over. They aren't collapsed. Why isn't that enough? He's still got a strong pulse at the wrist, so his blood pressure is still good. He's still got enough blood.

His pulse is fast. He is bleeding inside like a burst dam.

I quit the IV, mostly out of frustration. I must solve the breathing problem. I grab the stethoscope.

"Ron, keep bagging the guy."

Ron presses the oxygen in as fast as the bag will re-inflate. Full air sounds fill my ears. *What the hell is going on? He's getting air to his lungs. Why can't he breathe?*

I'll think about this while I try the IV again. The tourniquet still bands his arm. Nothing new popped up.

Damn.

"Scott, it's getting hard to bag."

I pull away from the man's arm again. The patient no longer fights. His eyes stare motionless at the ceiling and they glaze over. His chest no longer rises with any attempt to breathe. I glance at the heart monitor. His pulse rate is still clicking along at 140.

Shit. I can't keep up with this guy. Time to intubate.

I tear into the bag with the intubation equipment. I need to put a tube into the man's lungs so Ron can continue breathing for him. I rip open the package to one of the tubes, hook up a syringe and inflate the balloon on the other end. This tests the balloon to make sure it will hold air. I deflate the balloon, grab the laryngoscope handle and attach a curved blade. Wide and flat, it moves the tongue aside to view the vocal cords, the landmark for the procedure. I bring the blade to a 90-degree angle, turning on a light bulb at the end. The mouth is a dark place. I'm ready to go.

"Ron, move out of there. I've gotta intubate him."

We switch places. This puts me above the guy's head. I pull his lower lip down so I don't mash it all to hell. If this guy lives, no use giving him a fat lip.

I push on his jaw, intending to open his teeth, slip the blade in, lift his tongue, glimpse the vocal cords, and shove the tube into his lungs. His mouth doesn't move.

Shit. His jaw's clamped shut.

We swerve on that familiar turn into the hospital.

Out of time. Damn. He's not breathing, either.

"Ron, keep bagging him."

We switch places again. I pop the tourniquet off the guy's arm on my way by and put the heart monitor by the back doors as Bill comes around and whips them open. Ron yanks the oxygen tubing from the wall mount and throws it to me. I catch it, shove the end on a portable bottle and lay the bottle between the patient's legs. Bill waits, one hand on the end of the gurney, the other on the release and ready to push it the instant I give the go ahead.

I give a final scan to ensure we aren't going to tear anything off that's important to the patient or expensive, as we exit the ambulance.

"Okay, Bill. Clear."

The gurney's legs touch the ground and I say to everyone, "Go in easy, guys. Let's not dump him."

Catching a curb as we go in and flipping the gurney? That would be the shits.

We all move quickly into the emergency department. Bill and Ron drive the gurney. I bag the man as we roll into the trauma room full of people. Bill and I lift the patient on the backboard to the hospital gurney and a respiratory therapist takes over bagging. I step back and begin with a firm voice.

"We have an approximately thirty-year-old male with multiple gunshot wounds about his body."

The entire room listens to my report but everyone strains like a rubber band at its limit: taut and anxious to fly. My allowance of about thirty seconds steadily flakes away.

"From the top, he has one through and through to his left pinna; one in his right, central chest; one in his right arm continuing through to his right chest; a graze shot to his left upper arm; one in his left butt and one in his left thigh. The engine crew had him stripped and on the board when I got to him. I didn't roll him to check his back. Initially conscious, he stated difficulty breathing. His lungs are clear, bilaterally, heart rate of 140 sinus tach, strong radial pulse. En route, he degraded to skins diaphoretic and pale, decreased respiratory to currently apneic. He maintained a pulse of 140. I attempted oral intubation but failed due to his locked jaw. I was unable to start an IV."

I step aside and the entire room jumps to action. I roll the empty gurney out of the trauma room. I turn toward the ambulance bay and punch the wall plate to open the doors.

I punched the plate harder than was needed. But that's how it starts: the shift from robotic, all-knowing caregiver, to failure, back to being human. Now, all I see is the end of the gurney as I run away from my patient. I am leaving him to begin dulling the memory of his ragged breathing. I am no longer required to crawl inside his chest and visualize the carnage. He is finishing the dying he started in my ambulance and I am running away.

The skin on my face stretches tight and my vision curls in from the outside as the end of the gurney passes through the doors. The scream stuffed down since I first got on scene presses the threshold of my stomach, but I am too close to the hospital to let go.

My hands grip the gurney, guiding me away. If it was up to my heart, I would run down the street and let all that roils in my stomach come screeching out in a loud, sickening wail. But I trust my fingers to not let go of the gurney. I turn toward the ambulance as the scream rises like a burst pipe under pressure.

The doors lie gaped open, the refuse from our attempts strewn on the floor. I slam the gurney at the back of the ambulance. The scream is a rising geyser out of control, scorching my throat.

The burning fills my eyes and the tears roll out. I choke back a sob, stumble to the front seat and crawl inside. The heat washes over me and I let go.

I failed him! He was talking to me! When we met he was talking to me! I couldn't intubate him. I couldn't get him enough oxygen. I didn't give him enough. I couldn't even start the fucking IV! What the fuck did I do for this guy?! Nothing!

I sit in the front of the ambulance and let the tears flow.

"Excuse me."

I open my eyes. A doctor stands next to me, one of the doctors from inside.

"Someone said you were having trouble."

I nod my head. I wipe the tears from my face. "Yeah, I couldn't get anything done on the way in."

"I want to tell you there is nothing you could have done. He was too messed up. You did the best job possible."

"Thanks."

The doctor walks back in the hospital.

I sit in the front of the ambulance and wrap myself in the heated air of the afternoon. Like a soft cocoon, the weight and stifle surround me and slowly allow me to pull myself together. I don't move. I barely breathe. A tear runs down my cheek, its trail dries on my skin. I don't wipe it. I want to feel. I want to feel something. I want texture, but I start small: The dried streak of a tear.

I replay what I did, what I saw.

My patient was a guy with seven bullet holes in him, at least two of them critical. I remember my hand's motion over his body. I evaluate my progression, top to bottom. I had been efficient. We had gotten him off the street fast. Nothing had been missed.

I did my work on the way to the hospital. Ron had been fantastic help, gotten him oxygen and switched to the BVM when I asked. We had switched to the BVM because the non-rebreather mask wasn't enough. The patient needed more. He was still conscious, so I couldn't intubate him.

Could the guy have taken a tube while conscious?

God knows I couldn't. The proper sized tube for him equals my index finger. And to place it, I would have had to wrench his tongue out of the way. No, I was right to wait on the tube. It was bad luck his mouth locked on me when he needed the tube.

So, what about the lungs? I heard a lot of air moving in and out with his breathing.

There was nothing wrong with his lungs. They worked fine. The bullets thrashed too many arteries. The blood to carry the oxygen poured like several loose fire hoses into his chest cavity. We had gotten him to the hospital swiftly. We had done everything possible on the way in. There had been too much damage. That I couldn't fix.

To do my job I must find the problem. I have medicine to change it. But with trauma, speed is the answer. How fast can I put him under a surgeon's knife? That we had done.

The squawk of the radio brings me out of my reflection, the heat now uncomfortable and stifling. I have to decide. I can leave, just start walking, and never experience this again. I tell myself that option is always there.

No, I can't do that. I have the privilege of being the person others call when they need help. This guy needed my help, badly, and I had given him my best. I was smooth, efficient, calm, and precise. The crew working with me, fast and accurate.

This guy had seven bullets put inside him by another person. That was the problem handed to me, my partner, and the crew from the fire engine. The guy had died from those injuries. We hadn't failed him. The problem was bigger than we could turn.

The positive thing is, because of our guy, the next critical patient will meet a crew of emergency professionals who have been down this road before. We will give that next guy our best, topped with the lessons learned. That is a team of which I want to be a part.

I get the patient's name from the hospital staff and I put the response times for the call on the paperwork. We were on scene in four minutes. We had him in the hospital eight minutes later. Daryl Robert Preston died in six.

CHAPTER 13

Gregg Stafford

"Hey, Gregg! What's up, man?"

Gregg Stafford tripped and stumbled his way down the sidewalk. Someone called 911. Figured he needed help.

I stepped to the sidewalk and deduced the most common of his three drunken paths to calculate a meeting point.

Tall, lanky, and hovering at least six inches over me, with wild and uncombed brown hair, he ran into my gloved hands.

"Gregg, hold up. Let's talk."

"Hurumph." And he staggered left.

I adjusted. "Gregg, my man. Stop a minute."

My partner, Robert, pulled the gurney and angled the bed directly behind Gregg. If required, I only needed to give a little push and he would fall back onto the mattress. That technique, however, usually pissed people off, and regaining a positive conversation with a drunk guy takes effort. If I could make him sit down on his own, our meeting would go much smoother.

"Greg, stop trying to walk."

By this time I held a grasp on his upper arm.

"Gregg, sit down before you fall down."

With a little pressure to his arm, not so much a push, I suggested to his alcohol-muddled brain a new direction of travel which happened to end on my gurney. Gregg sat, well, sort of crashed backwards, and his arms flew out to catch himself.

I successfully dodged.

"Well done, Gregg. Thank you."

Purposefully moving faster than Gregg's mind operated in this state, Robert and I soon had him buckled in and rolling to the ambulance.

"Hey, what the fucphgmn . . . ?"

"Yeah, Gregg. I hear you. You're staggering a bit much. Scaring the peoples. We're taking you to the hospital."

"Spiddlefiguskin."

"Yes, I feel the same."

The gurney got locked in and I followed to sit on the bench seat.

"So, Gregg, which hospital do you want to go to today?"

"Umscullentionally."

"Right. I'm guessing the closest one from here. Can I borrow your arm to take a blood pressure?"

"Fuck youllmskun."

"Now, Gregg, we're going to be polite."

I wrapped the cuff around his left arm and pumped it up, listening with my stethoscope for the beat of his pulse as I slowly let the air out.

The shift of his body gave me warning. Gregg's right fist came around searching for my head.

I ducked, grabbed Gregg's swinging arm and helped continue its path around his head, past his left ear, then forced his upper arm to tighten under his chin.

"Now, Gregg. I said we're going to be polite."

His body relaxed and I knew the fighting was ended.

"We'll have no more of that."

I released his arm and turned to Robert who was writing down the basic info about Gregg we both had memorized.

"All right, Robert. Saint Closest Hospital, if you will."

And that's how many of the transports went involving Gregg Stafford.

Other times Gregg was quite the good-natured guy.

"Hey, Gregg! What's up?"

"Awww, not feeling it today."

Now, to appreciate the proper picture of Gregg, beyond his wild hair and overall tallness, one had to experience him in conversation. Gregg spoke like every bad surfer actor in every bad movie about surfing. He also spoke loudly, with punctuation and hand gestures for emphasis. He was a lot of fun to watch and listen to.

"So, Gregg, what's bothering you?"

His voice filled the ambulance.

"My stomach, man. Hurts like a motherfucker."

"Sorry. When was the last time you ate a meal not involving a dumpster?"

"Yeah, been a while on that one, dude."

He sat back and smiled, like I'd guessed his secret.

"Vomiting and diarrhea?"

"Yup. Been putting it out both ends, man."

A solid declaration, with hand motions to match.

"Any blood from either one?"

"Naw. Just the squirts and been puking my guts out."

"All right. We'll run you on in. Got a preference which hospital today?"

"Nope. One I haven't pissed off lately." Sheepish smile.

"Saint Closest it is."

Another day I asked Gregg what his story was. Every unhoused guy has one because they all come from somewhere. Sometimes mental illness crowds out the memories and is the reason they can't pull it together enough to step off the streets. Other times alcohol or drugs cloud everything up and they never rid themselves of the haze.

Gregg looked at me while sitting on my gurney as we rode to the hospital, this time for chest pain, probably bronchitis, his face framed by that mane of wild brown hair.

"Well," he began, his raspy voice filling the ambulance. "I was born in Germany. Dad was in the Army. Then ... 1971 ... BOOM! Good 'ol U S of A! Went to Johnson High. Graduated. Been fucking around ever since."

Gregg graduated high school, woke up on Monday, and simply did ... nothing. Tuesday he woke up and ... did nothing, again. Ten years later he was in my ambulance. But it was another day, a few years ago, that explains why I remember Gregg.

"Medic 62 respond, Code 2, to Second Street cross of E Street for the fall."

The problem was clear from a block away. Gregg had found a bicycle, a prized possession in the unhoused community, but was staggering.

I stepped out of the ambulance.

"Afternoon, Gregg. Nice bike."

He was sporting a little scrape on his forehead.

"How'd you get the scrape?"

"Must have fallen down. It ain't bothering me none."

"Let me check you out real quick."

I took hold of both sides of his head and ran my fingers firmly down the back of his neck.

"Does that hurt?"

"No, man. I'm fine."

I continued by running my fingers down the middle of his back, pressing on the vertebrae as I went. He staggered a bit, showing he was maintaining his usual level of drunk.

"How about that? Does that hurt?"

"Nope. I'm telling you, man. I'm all good today."

"All right. You seem like you're with it. Do you want to go to the hospital?"

"No."

I don't know why I gave him the choice. It seemed all right that day.

"Don't ride the bike. Walk from here."

"Okay, dude."

He gave an enthusiastic thumbs up.

Gregg walked away from me. Ten feet later he swung his leg over the seat and started off.

"Damn," I said to Robert. "Let's go get him."

We pulled ahead and I jumped out.

"Gregg, you're too drunk for this. Don't ride your bike. If you ride your bike, I'm going to have to call the cops."

"All right. I won't."

And he walked away just to climb back on again a few feet down the sidewalk.

We drove up to him but this time he wouldn't stop.

Gregg now had his own personal ambulance following him as he weaved on his bicycle. He shifted over to the street and took a right turn. We followed. Gregg's foot slipped off the pedal, causing him to pitch left. He stayed upright. His foot slipped off the right pedal and he pitched right. Gregg was doing acrobatics on his bike I couldn't do sober.

Gregg signaled with his left arm up, bent at the elbow. The Department of Motor Vehicles would have been proud of his textbook presentation of a right turn signal. He then took a left turn onto Third Street. This portion is three lanes wide, one for each direction and a center turn lane.

Gregg pedaled and swerved his way using all three lanes. We had our emergency lights flashing and, thankfully, alert drivers slowed and avoided his path as we cruised along. The street takes a dip to go underneath the shopping mall and Gregg hunkered down over the handlebars to speed down the hill toward a shelter four blocks away. A cop, who had apparently happened upon our whole show, pulled in between us. I yelled out the window.

"His name's Gregg!"

The cop called out on his PA system for Gregg to stop. Gregg's pedaling never faltered and I almost heard his voice in my head and knew what he was thinking.

"Dude, if I can just make it to the shelter, I'll be fine."

Robert and I made a left turn.

CHAPTER 14

Berwick Slader

"Hey, Scott. We would like you to take on a paramedic student." The local program director called and she wanted to chat. "The student we want to give you? Well, don't be afraid to fail him."

"No problem. That is my attitude when I teach."

If the student doesn't meet the standard, they flunk. They must pass me to become a paramedic. Many of us call it the grandmother test. Would you feel comfortable having your student work on your grandmother?

"His name is Berwick Slader."

I had never heard of a Berwick before.

"He came to us and wanted to be an EMT. He took our course and he passed. He did well."

"Yeah, go on."

"After EMT school, he said he wanted to go straight into paramedic school."

Little bells started going off in my head. I had been down this road. I slammed my way through the two levels of EMT and to paramedic in slightly over one year. Partly because of that I dropped back to an EMT for four years and retook paramedic school.

Berwick was barreling down the same path and not taking "no" for an answer.

The director relented and told him, "Okay. We'll let you in the school. You'll never get past the book portion." Berwick did. "You passed. You'll never complete the hospital portion." Berwick did. "This last part is the toughest. You won't survive the paramedic portion. You must function to the satisfaction of a working paramedic."

The jobs of EMT and paramedic build on each other. As an EMT you learn how to look at a patient, how to do a basic physical exam, and about the tools you have at the

EMT level to make a difference. The paramedic learns about the body systems and how things break. It is a more in-depth study. You get the tools and permitted skills to fix a broader range of problems with a greater chance of catastrophic failure. The paramedic who never did the work as an EMT must learn both the observational exercises of the EMT and the advanced problem-solving questions of the medic at the same time. The director knew that was a tall order.

"Scott, don't be afraid to fail him."

"I won't. He has to meet my standards or I will fail him."

Then I met him. Berwick was not the typical rescuer, going-to-save-your-daughter type. Tall and gangly, he wore big, black-framed glasses and a wide, quirky smile. Always grinning, he reminded me of a Labrador retriever. *"Throw me the stick. I'll go get the stick."*

No problem. He's outta here.

On the first day I do introductions.

"In the beginning I'm doing all the work and you're watching. In the end you're doing all the work, I'm reading the newspaper and getting paid."

Obviously, a lot more stress boils up on both sides. I am charged with creating a functioning paramedic in a short time while the student converts all the book material just learned into real life experiences. And in the meantime, the patients don't slow down on dying.

I tell all my interns, "Don't worry about the patient. They will be treated and treated well. But if things go sideways, make sure you're in the ambulance when I'm ready to go. I will leave you."

So, Berwick and I began our Summer of Love and strange things happened. I found Berwick would actually listen to what I said. He accepted criticism and changed his behavior. I grew to like Berwick. He was goofy, for sure, but I had a goofy sense of humor. He cared about people. I loved taking care of people. He was anxious to learn. I loved teaching people about my job. We were a perfect fit.

Besides the medical skills a paramedic student must absorb, there were personality traits I, as a preceptor, must foster. A paramedic must be in charge. He or she must be able to step forward and direct a small cadre of other professionals while also ensuring the family is kept calm and informed of their loved one's condition. The onset of this condition may be the most dramatic thing this family has experienced and/or the medical crew may walk in and get hit with the biggest gut punch of a scenario. The paramedic must carry on… with confidence.

Paramedics and their partners must also ensure a top-notch working environment in a world where things are constantly moving and shifting. The polite term is to be fastidious. A paramedic must be insane about doing it right, doing it right all the time, and finding the nitpicky things. Fine. A touch of OCD is not a bad thing. Anyway, these were traits my preceptors developed in me and important traits to bring forward in Berwick.

As an example, I began my day by checking my ambulance. I rode the same ambulance and counted the same stuff I inventoried the previous morning. Maybe someone used my ambulance after I left and forgot to replace something or my partner and I forgot something as we locked up the night before. That's one of the hard things about being a paramedic: To pore over the same equipment at the beginning of every shift, twenty-four hours after the last time I checked, and make sure the counts are correct and everything works, requires stamina. Again, possessing those personal qualities served me well with a patient in front of me. For instance, Cereal Time.

I ate breakfast before I went to work. I got hungry about eleven o'clock and tolerated my hunger until noon. However, the EMS Gods liked to play games with those of us who tried to make plans or set a schedule while on the clock and invariably they would toss me a call just before I dug out my sandwich. I was trying to watch my girlish figure, so if I ate a healthy snack mid-morning, the call out of the blue wouldn't throw off my whole day.

Cereal Time was at ten-thirty and non-negotiable. I would pour the milk and eat while riding along at sixty miles per hour on a country road.

Lately, I liked Frosted Mini-Wheats. I liked the "crunchy on one side and sugar on the other side" thing. I brought a container with the cereal, a Thermos with milk and a spoon. Cereal Time. Ten-thirty.

Our ambulance served as our work space, transportation, classroom, and break room twelve hours a day, four days a week. I went to the cabinet where we stored our personal gear and pulled out my cereal container. I got the cooler holding the milk and the spoon. I opened the container.

Hey, these are Corn Flakes.

I peered into the depths of the cabinet but found no other container. In fact, the container appeared to be mine. I looked again. Corn Flakes. I scanned the cabinet. No, it was the only one.

Yes, they are Corn Flakes.

Corn Flakes were not Frosted Mini-Wheats. I loved Frosted Mini-Wheats. Corn Flakes would do, but they didn't have that crunchy on one side and sugar on the other side thing going for them. I mean I could eat Corn Flakes, but they weren't Frosted Mini-Wheats. Berwick stood behind me while I filled with angst.

Where are my Mini-Wheats?

In fact, I didn't think I had Corn Flakes in my house. Where did these come from?

Over the shock of missing my Mini-Wheats, I resigned myself to eating Corn Flakes. However, now there was a mystery to solve. I loved mysteries, a fine trait to have as a paramedic. A paramedic always needed to ask and keep asking, "Why?"

So, where did these Corn Flakes come from?

Yeah, Berwick switched the cereal.

Berwick and I had fun in other ways. Each day I walked in and, with my best drill sergeant's voice, I hollered, "Berwick! Drop and give me twenty in the name of EMS!"

Berwick would reply, "Yes, sir! One a day for the next twenty days, Sir!"

Never did get one push-up out of him.

On other days he struggled with the mountain of information being tossed at him. I gave him words of encouragement and reminded him, "If you really don't feel you can continue, I want you to learn this phrase: "Do you want fries with that?'"

In our ambulance, the cab and the back were blocked off from each other. A little window was cut between the two spaces where someone could see forward and talk to those up front. Berwick lived there for two months.

One day he filled the window and professed with his goofy smile, "Hey, it's the intern channel. No options and no commercials."

Berwick did progress in his internship. Early in his training we walked in on a patient complaining of shortness of breath. I gave Berwick about ten seconds to push things in the right direction. He didn't.

Dave and I jumped in, got her some oxygen, gave her a breathing treatment, and hustled her into the ambulance.

On another day we parked outside a convenience store. We were experts at knowing the local eateries and places with shade, depending on the time of day. We got a call for abdominal pain and drove to the house.

We got out but Berwick didn't. Berwick didn't because he wasn't there. After we didn't need the fire engine and their medical assistance anymore, I pulled the officer aside.

"Hey, can you do me a favor? My intern is back at that little shopping center around the corner. Would you mind picking him up?"

Berwick's version of the story was, "I stepped out to buy a soda. When I came out, you guys were gone. I said to myself, 'Oh well, they'll come back for me at some point. I might as well sit down on this bench and wait.' Then this fire engine comes around the corner and waves me over. They say to get in. I have never ridden in a fire engine before. It was so cool."

Yeah.

"Berwick, next time, tell me when you step out of the ambulance."

The interesting thing about the call was this lady's severe abdominal pain. She also had a huge belly. Not like pregnant huge, but a hard ball right around the navel. I didn't have a clue. The ball didn't pulsate but hurt her when I pushed on it. The doctor drained out about two liters of urine. She really had to go to the bathroom.

Berwick's biggest call came at the end of his internship when a man tripped over a cord on the roof and fell off.

We arrived on scene and one of the firefighters met us on the sidewalk. He is a paramedic and I've known him for years. He said, "Hey, Scott, this guy's bad. We've got to move on this one."

The fire guys already had him packaged on a backboard, the neck brace in place: he was taped to the board. Berwick took a look. The man's face was a bloody mess after landing on his head and hitting cement.

"Scott, I want to intubate this guy."

Everyone turned to me. The firefighters saw the patient needed a surgeon most of all. But I also knew when to validate my student's decisions.

"Berwick, you've got thirty seconds—and one try."

Intubation does two things: One, it helps them breathe. Two, emesis is prevented from going into the guy's lungs if he throws up while he is strapped on his back.

Berwick pulled out the equipment, opened the blade attached to a handle, placed the curved blade between the man's lips and lifted his tongue. By doing this, a paramedic can pinpoint the vocal cords, the landmark, and put the tube straight into the trachea. The procedure is made easier by raising the shoulders and tipping the head back. It is a tense skill, but with practice it can be done relatively easily. The fall and obvious trauma to this man's head changed all that. Berwick had to attempt his intubation without moving the guy's neck and while peering through a bloody mess.

After a few seconds Berwick gave up, pulled out the blade and said, "It's dark in there. Let's move."

A good paramedic knows when to do a procedure and, sometimes more importantly, when to give up and change direction. I was proud of him. Berwick made the exact decision I would have.

We had the man at the hospital in seven minutes.

I found out later that a few minutes before the man fell, a pile of insulation had been removed that might have lessened the impact. I still see that patient walking around town. He had a rough time for a while. He lost a lot in his life, but he works and can drive his truck again. We did good things for him.

A few days after that call, I went to a local fast food restaurant and picked up a job application. On our next shift, we drove to the hospital where both the doctor in charge of the paramedic program and the director of the program, the charge nurse for that day, were working. I handed the restaurant application to the doctor.

The doctor called us all to come to the office. He looked sternly at Berwick and said, "You are near the end of your internship. Here are two forms. I want you to tell me which one you deserve." He handed Berwick the job application and his final, successful, evaluation. Berwick scanned the top form, which contained the restaurant logo as a watermark in background relief printed as large as the paper.

Berwick began mumbling the first question aloud, "How far do you live from the restaurant?" He continued to read the application while the rest of us in the room struggled to keep from laughing.

He twisted his face in confusion as he tried to understand what he was reading. He finally saw the logo in background relief, remembered he could have chosen the phrase "Do you want fries with that?" as a training alternative, and his face spread into his huge quirky grin. We all broke out laughing and congratulated Berwick on successfully completing his paramedic internship. He beat the odds and defied all who had not believed he could do it.

Berwick is still a paramedic. I keep tabs on him. He has become a supervisor and is described as a good paramedic. He was involved in a shift bid and was required to present a written request for his preference — which he submitted on a six-foot-long piece of butcher paper and in crayon replete with pretty colors, fanciful designs, and childish English. Berwick never did anything the right way.

Then again, in solving problems and taking care of patients, is there just one right way? And the medic who digs for some hidden symptom or devises a wildly creative idea to free the patient who is pinned beneath a car, isn't that the medic I want treating my grandmother?

CHAPTER 15

If You Can Do It Better

I thought I was handling the whole pregnancy thing pretty well. Camille was healthy, things were progressing as they should; she's a nurse and I'm a medic. We had wholehearted support from our families, we loved our doctor. I was ready to open up to this new bundle of joy.

I just needed to finish this shift.

After today I had two weeks off. Camille and I made an appointment at the hospital in three days if "things" didn't commence, after which I began to, well, you know, raise a kid. I already had an eight-year-old who came with the wife as a package deal. Justine had taught me a lot about the role of Daddy and I felt suited, but I started with her at age three. This was my first foray into infantdom.

Twelve hours to go.

Dave and I went to a call for a "man down." We pulled up to the house and I tripped getting out of the ambulance. I recovered and started toward the front door of the house.

Dave's calm voice floated in from behind me.

"I'll bring all the stuff by myself. You go ahead."

"Oh, sorry."

I turned back and grabbed my share of equipment.

The fire engine arrived and the five of us were led by a lady to the living room. A man, about eighty, lay on the bare hardwood floor in a puddle of his urine wearing only a thin t-shirt and his underwear.

I asked the lady, "How long has he been on the floor?"

"I don't know. I'm his daughter. We call him every few days to check on him. Last time I talked to him was two days ago. This morning I called and he didn't answer the phone. I came right over and found him on the floor."

"So he may have been down for two days?"

"Um, yes. It's possible."

"Okay. What's his name?"

"Lowe. James Lowe."

Dave took the clipboard, shepherded the daughter to somewhere else in the house and questioned her about her father, his condition, and what she had seen. Dave was also to gather and list the medications.

I dropped my bags nearby.

What's first?

On a usual day, a list of to-dos would flow out and I'd begin passing out duties, but not this morning.

Vital signs are always a fine place to start.

I flipped open my kit, pulled out the stethoscope and blood pressure cuff, and knelt at Mr. Lowe's right side.

"Hello, sir. My name is Scott. I'm a paramedic and we're going to get you out of here."

I watched for any sign of recognition in his eyes, something saying he'd heard me and understood. Nothing. I poked his arm. No reaction. I then rubbed a knuckle in his chest. This is a test for deep unconsciousness using painful stimuli. Mr. Lowe's eyes focused on me, his hand grabbed toward mine, and he mumbled, "Ouch! Piss off, Rachel!"

"Sir, I'm the paramedic. Are you in pain?"

"Rachel, are you home now?"

Most likely dehydrated, dangerously cold, and hungry. I declared Mr. Lowe confused, localizing pain with stimuli.

Moving on with my assessment, I counted a pulse off his wrist, did the math to arrive at ninety-two beats per minute, then wrapped the blue cloth of the blood pressure cuff around his arm. The cuff hung sloppy because his upper arm branched from his shoulder as little more than bone. I plugged my ears with my stethoscope, placed it at the crease of his elbow, and strained to catch the faint beats of his blood pressure. A soft voice from behind me excused its way through my concentration.

"Hey, um, Scott. Do you want to put this guy on the monitor?"

It was Matt, the EMT from the fire engine. He had asked if I wanted a continuous visual readout of his pulse and heart activity, which might give a clue if an irregular heartbeat caused him to fall. Excellent suggestion.

"Yeah, thanks, Matt. Let's do that."

I turned back to my blood pressure and attempts to create a to-do list. Matt placed stickers on our patient's chest.

"Hey, Scott. Do you want this guy on oxygen?"

My mind snapped away from the blood pressure — again.

Wow, another fantastic idea. Confusion can be caused by a lack of oxygen to the brain. The brain, if experiencing a stroke, can benefit from extra oxygen. Definitely.

"Yes, Matt. Good idea. Thanks. Please put him on a mask at ten liters per minute."

Back to my attempts while Matt strapped a mask over our man's face.

Focus. Just finish one thing. I've taken this guy's pulse. It's not too fast or too slow. Get this blood pressure, then figure out what to do next.

"Hey, Scott."

What! I wanted to say, but that would have been wrong.

Matt, as an EMT "assisting" the paramedic, was doing a fantastic job caring for this patient. He continued.

"Do you want to put this guy in cervical precautions?"

Did I want to protect this man's spine from any possible injury he may have suffered from his fall? Since the patient acted confused and unable to help us, Matt's suggestion was yet another terrific idea.

"Yes, Matt. Let's do cervical precautions."

And he left to gather the equipment for that procedure.

Time for me to wake up. Dave was off gathering information and a medications list; I had been fumbling with a blood pressure, which I finally heard at one hundred and thirty over seventy. By God, Matt was the only one actually treating the patient. I didn't know where I was, but I had not been in this man's living room.

After Matt, the rest of the fire crew and I got the man packaged; I yelled to Dave we were ready to leave. Dave appeared and helped us wrangle the patient out of the house and into the ambulance.

I planned the rest of my treatment as we pulled away. First I needed to check Mr. Lowe's blood sugar level. Then I should start an IV, the treatment for a confused, dehydrated person who possibly suffered from exposure while lying on his floor. I also began to gather my thoughts for our arrival at the hospital. I would need the information Dave had gotten.

"Hey, Dave," I yelled up front. "Where's the clipboard?"

"Damn, I put it down in the living room to help you guys out the door."

Another stumble among stumbles already too numerous on this call. Yes, Dave carried the clipboard inside the house. But, as the team leader, all responsibility for the flow and outcome fell to me.

A lot of this job is the appearance of knowing what one is doing and prioritizing. Going back to the house to pick up my forgotten clipboard would delay the care of our patient. Any action that didn't improve his health was not important. Carry on. Time to start an IV.

I roped up his arm with the tourniquet to make the veins stand out. Nothing. I kept searching in hopes something would pop up. I let his arm hang to let the blood pool a little. A hint of something rose as a suggestion in the bend of his elbow. Maybe I could get that vein.

I prepped everything and stuck the catheter in his arm. Nothing. No flashback, no blood flowing into the back of the catheter. I fished around a little. Still nothing. Oh well. This IV wasn't essential. It was only a new hole in his arm and about twenty-five cc's of salt water run in before we got to the hospital. Starting it was more of a courtesy to the nurses.

I could still get something out of this. I had to do a check of his sugar and I needed one drop of blood. I popped the tourniquet and pressed on his arm above the catheter to prevent any spray as I withdrew the needle, turned and dropped it into the sharps container. As I leaned away, I released my grip on his vein. I wanted to let him bleed a little, draw my sample and then clean up.

I picked up the glucometer for my sugar check and turned back to find no blood. He didn't leak a drop. I squeezed the hole I made with the large needle. Nothing. I moved his arm around and fiddled and prodded. I couldn't pull a drop out of this guy. I truly missed the entire vein when looking for the IV. Well, that sucked.

We pulled into the hospital. Great. It was time to unload and present my patient, starting with a verbal report, to the professional staff of the emergency department where I went several times every shift I worked.

We got inside and transferred our patient over to the hospital gurney. I readied myself to speak, usually done with my clipboard as a reference. Not this time. Wonderful. The nurse waited as I struggled with where to begin on my ordinarily fluid presentation. Then the doctor decided to wander in as well. I swallowed hard.

"We bring you an approximately eighty-year old man (I couldn't remember his birth date), a Mister James Lowe (I at least remembered that much). Mr. Lowe's daughter found him on his living room floor down for an unknown amount of time, maybe up to two days. She'll be coming to the hospital soon (I couldn't even trot out a reliable family member as a source of information). He is confused verbally, unknown if that is his normal state, but he responds to painful stimuli appropriately. He is incontinent of urine. His vital signs are a pulse of ninety-two and a blood pressure of one hundred and thirty over seventy. Respirations are non-labored at sixteen. His skins are cool but dry and of good color. Lungs are clear."

This is where things got dicey. I relied on the hope they knew me and were well aware I normally did better than what I was about to plunge into. Big breath.

"We forgot the clipboard at the scene and on that clipboard is his birth date and his medicines." Sheepish grin. "I also tried to start an IV on the way in. I missed."

I scanned my audience to evaluate the success of my little soft-shoe routine. So far no exasperation. And now for the finish.

"And, while I was going to give you his blood sugar, I couldn't even pull a drop out of this man." I wanted to end on a positive note. "But, I did put him on the heart monitor. That looked normal. He is on oxygen and he is in spinal precautions because of his altered state and unwitnessed fall (all thanks to Matt)."

Big smile. Ta da!

The nurse and doctor both shook their heads and saw right through my act.

I went and got a fresh chart out of the stash we carried in the ambulance. Dave filled in the staff on what he remembered from his conversation with the daughter at the house. Later, I pulled Dave aside and told him of my problems with patient management.

"Dave, you and I are both medics. This is my last day before I take off and go have a baby — sort of. Would you mind taking the patients today? Can I just drive? I'm not into this and I don't trust myself."

"Sure Scott. I'll see you through."

"Thanks."

And off we went to find someone still at the patient's home to retrieve our clipboard.

Later that day we were assigned a transfer. A patient needed to go from one hospital to another, but she was sick enough we needed one of our company nurses to do the patient care. Dave and I were to be his assistant and driver.

Sweet.

Dave was going to drive and Ben was going to do patient care. I planned on hiding behind the patient and assuming no responsibility. Everyone was safe. We went, got our patient, and loaded her in.

Our tires left the driveway of the first hospital, three miles from the second hospital, and our lady spoke to Ben sitting at her elbow.

"I'm having chest pain."

This was not what we hoped to hear during our short transport. The heart monitor sat on a small rack behind the patient's head, pointed at me, and merrily tracing the electrical impulses radiating from her heart.

Ben looked at me. He was a terrific nurse but needed information to develop a treatment plan.

"Scott, what does the monitor say?"

I had fully settled into my role of quiet observer. I saw the monitor and I could easily read it. I also understood we had progressed beyond a simple three-mile transfer from hospital to hospital.

I decoded the green blip trailing a line across the screen. The blip bounced up and down in a normal manner, all the bumps and points in their correct places. All the spaces between those points were correct. Ah, wait a minute. The back segment of the Q-wave no longer went back down to the middle. In fact, it stayed all the way to the top and carried straight into the T-wave. This was not good. That elevated S-T segment or, more importantly, its rocketing change from the path the tracing followed just a moment ago, clearly stated our patient was having a heart attack—now. I needed to relay this finding to Ben, who calmly waited for my interpretation.

"There are . . . there are some . . . changes," I stammered.

"What kind of changes," he said through clenched teeth.

"Um, well."

And that was about as far as I got. Ben reached over and flipped the monitor to face him. He swiftly read the problem and understood its meaning.

"Ma'am. Are you having chest pain right now?"

"Yes, it is really crushing."

Ben glared back at me as I sat in a near catatonic state. He jumped across the ambulance and grabbed the medication kit stored above my head.

Again, through clenched teeth, "Fine. I'll give the nitro."

We got her to the hospital. She died three hours later.

I felt an eerie sensation. I had been talking to this woman and now my name appeared on the list of people who spoke to her last. I was also angry — at myself. A patient had been in my ambulance, I had not been totally on my game, and she died. I was completely confident I didn't slow Ben down enough to cause or contribute to her death. Besides, the reason for the transport was her unstable cardiac condition. But, if I had been in charge of this woman, I couldn't be absolutely sure I would have acted quickly and with surety. That was unacceptable.

I did survive to the end of the shift without any more problems. I left Dave and the ambulance for a few weeks off work so I could focus on my wife and experience the wonder of childbirth as a father and not a caregiver.

Three days later I made camp in the delivery room with Camille. I was there for every contraction and under Camille's direction, counting how long each lasted and pushing my fist into the small of her back to take the pain down a notch. And I was there to deliver our perfect, beautiful child into the world.

CHAPTER 16

Dinner Time, Ambulance Style

After nine years working in Sonoma County, it was time to change jobs. I felt no desire to move further up the food chain and I was already on the busiest ambulance in the county. Thirty-two years old and confined to the right front seat for, conceivably, another thirty years didn't work for me. I loved the people I worked with, but I didn't see myself doing exactly the same job with little desirable advancement for that long—which brought me again to the San Francisco Department of Public Health, Paramedic Division.

A new job in a whole new city with many exciting chances for advancement seemed like a smart move. I would be doing the same job, picking up people with their problem of the day, but I'd be in San Francisco. Because of the population difference, 150,000 versus up to 1.5 million, the odds of something crazy or fantastically weird happening quadrupled. If that weird thing was going to happen, I wanted to be in the middle of it. Also, in a few months, the Paramedic Division would be transitioning over to the Fire Department.

That seemed like a wise thing for my career path. But I worried about that later because, first, there was tons to learn. I had to memorize the major street layout of a densely populated city built on seven hills and the traffic corridors to navigate from here to ten hospitals, while proving my ability as a paramedic. I gained a bonus from doing half my paramedic training in San Francisco. Now I was expected to be a top-notch paramedic in a system that didn't slow down for anybody and spit out casualties without blinking. Oh, and I got assigned the night shift.

My shift started at 1900 hours, seven p.m. for the non-initiated, and ended at 0700 hours three days a week,

Friday, Saturday, and Sunday. I still lived in Santa Rosa, which meant a one-hour drive home, pack in six hours of sleep and two hours to shower, shave, and kiss Camille and the kids before getting in the car for a repeat cycle. Every other Monday I would end the shift at seven in the morning, then be scheduled nine hours later for another shift until midnight. On those days I slept in the bunkroom above the station, woke, showered, and found something to eat before going back on duty. My wife didn't like the schedule much and I wasn't hot about night shift, but I loved the increased excitement, the newness of working in a huge city and being a part of San Francisco.

At first, I bounced around, filling in when someone's partner went on vacation or called in sick. Eventually, I was assigned to work with James.

James was, like me, in his early thirties. Thin, with a continuous three-day collection of unshaven blonde scruff, his uniform pulled from the floorboard of his car and his mouth from the closest sewer. A month or so into our partnership, I noticed he occasionally shook his boot while walking. It turned out James did have a soft side. He collected a few coins and kept them in his right boot in tribute to his grandfather who had done the same thing. Beyond that little tidbit, I found his persona to be an acquired taste and eloquence was not his strong point.

Our latest patient lay on the gurney and James sat in the jump seat above the patient's head, filling in the perfunctory data on the patient care report. I undressed the guy and passed information to James found via a wallet biopsy.

"If you don't hurry up with this fucker, I'm going to resort to peeing into a glove."

I didn't believe he would, but James had his own way of saying he was ready to go the hospital.

"Hold on. I'm trying to find a blood pressure."

"Don't worry about the blood pressure. I already wrote one-thirty-two over sixty-eight on the PCR."

James was kidding. He may cut a lot of corners but he never falsified information or compromised patient care with his laissez-faire façade.

I finished up the pressure and ripped off the cuff.

"One-forty over seventy-eight. Okay, let's go. I'll do the rest on the way to the hospital. Then I need food."

James handed the clipboard over to me and stepped out the side door. Before he pushed it closed he said,

"Yeah, right. Good luck."

James started toward the hospital while I sat back and worked on finishing the PCR by our arrival. Dispatch gave us twenty minutes to finish paperwork. If I turned it in early and we didn't tell anyone, we used that time to search out some quick food.

We'd been busting our butts ever since the shift started and Dispatch didn't care, the calls sat backed up on their screen and holding for an hour. We were an inanimate ambulance taking calls off their board and onto our log sheet. At the rate of one call an hour, our little joke resonated like that ad for nuts, "A call an hour, that's all we ask." The problem was, most calls took around an hour to run from dispatch to completion. My stomach just about declared a work stoppage.

I could have chosen to bring my food in a little cooler. I did cooler food in Santa Rosa. My capabilities, however, extended to bread, sliced meat, cheese, and mustard. I might branch out into a yogurt, which meant packing a spoon. I also did carrots and celery.

Some created sumptuous delicacies rising from the plastic confines of Tupperware.

"Just a little something left over from dinner last night."

"I like deli meat on rye four days a week."

No, I didn't.

And why didn't Camille make me lunch and send me out the door with a kiss like Betty Crocker? I had not married Betty Crocker. Camille was busy working at the hospital; caring for two kids, one a toddler; pregnant with our third child; and thinking that at one time she had a husband who helped around the house. No, I was left to fend for myself.

San Francisco is a culinary smorgasbord. Pick your gastronomic country and you can find it there. I once ate a Philly Cheese Steak sandwich at an Italian restaurant owned by Koreans. Eating in the ambulance, however, was a skill that limited how, when, and what type of food we were permitted to enjoy. My choice for the day needed to be ready in a few minutes and portable. Even during consumption, the meal might have to be packed up in seconds. It became quite limiting. For example, soup was tough.

We had turned over care of our patient to the incredibly tolerant nurses of the emergency department. How they avoided going crazy when they dealt with belligerent drunks every night, every shift, was hard to see. James was outside prepping the gurney and I was sitting inside at the nurses' station, putting the final flourishes on another stellar PCR when my radio crackled.

"Eighty-eight."

My stomach dropped and I looked at my watch. We had been at the hospital for ten minutes. *Damn.*

I keyed up the mike. "Eighty-eight. Francis. Paperwork."

Telling Dispatch I still had paperwork was my only option to try and steal a few minutes back. Blatantly whining over the airwaves only pissed them off and gave the rest of the eavesdropping ambulance fleet ammunition for the next two weeks.

"Yeah, sorry eighty-eight. Can you clear? We've got another one like you just brought in a few blocks away."

I fought back the anger. I wanted some food!

Then I heard James answer up, his voice almost chipper.

"Eighty-eight. Copy. Where to?"

What?! James knew we needed dinner. He hadn't even discussed it with me before accepting the call. I grabbed the clipboard and huffed outside.

"What the hell? I'm hungry here."

"Cool your God-damned jets. We're scoring dinner on this one. It's your turn to drive. Jump the fuck in."

I pulled away from the curb and pointed the ambulance toward Eddy and Leavenworth, the location of our next drunk guy, while James began his instruction.

"The beauty of this call," James instructed as I swung a right turn, "is we have a lot of opportunity to direct this patient's future. So, drive to the Thai Café on Geary and Leavenworth. Go in and order our dinner; I'm having the Pad Thai. We scrape up this drunk son of a bitch and grab our dinner on the way back to the hospital."

In my naiveté about how this works I asked, "But what if the patient wants to go to a hospital in the other direction from the restaurant?"

James shot me a look. "Shut the fuck up and drive."

After placing our dinner order and driving the remaining three blocks, we arrived at Eddy and Leavenworth. Our patient lay sprawled on the sidewalk nearly unconscious from his life of inebriation. The brilliance and simplicity of our plan became clear and I now understood why James eagerly snagged this call. He recognized we would get dinner by taking this very call. Remaining available left it to the whims of the Ambulance Gods whether we would actually get dinner and any other type of call was a crap shoot for our hospital destination.

We rolled our John Doe onto a flat stretcher, put him in the ambulance, and did the required vitals, sugar check, and physical exam. I jumped in the front, threw the shifter into drive, headed back to the Thai Café, got out, grabbed our dinner and laid it on the floor between the front seats.

Food never went in the back, at least not without four layers of sterility laid down beforehand. And the inverse stated no patient care activity or articles of use ever came to the front of the ambulance. The front was our sanctuary and not to be defiled.

The aromas of James' Pad Thai and my chow mein filled the ambulance. I could almost taste it and so could my stomach. It was not hard to imagine. I had eaten this same dish four days ago.

I pulled to the curb in front of the same hospital I left twenty-two minutes before and finished delivering our patient for his umpteenth rehabilitation from a drunken stupor. I reassembled the ambulance, then ate my dinner in the remaining seven minutes before James completed the paperwork and walked outside. James downed his as we drove to the next call.

On another day James showed me the proper way to eat the chicken dinner from a restaurant on 21st and Folsom. First I donned gloves. Eating with gloves on was standard, which removed a lot of the worry about getting messy. In fact, it allowed me to be messy. If we got a call, strip the gloves, close the lid, and we're off to the races.

This delectable meal was chicken breasts spiced to perfection and served with rice, beans, sauce, and tortillas. Instructed to rip the chicken from the bone, I created a mish-mash with all the other ingredients. Once mixed, load some on a tortilla and eat. Delicious and portable. The same goes for burritos. It's the same dinner but wrapped in a tortilla, then wrapped in foil. Just peel down and eat.

Another problem was our shift hours. James and I worked night shift. San Francisco may be a major metropolitan city but most restaurants close by eleven—only four hours into our twelve-hour shift. Well, there really was no problem if we ignored the food storage rules and didn't mind eating the other half of the burrito rolling in its foil and sitting on the floor for five hours.

I've gotten good at making meals disappear. I can clear a plate of almost any food product in moments and still have time to properly use a napkin. My wife knows this. She reminds me quite often as I sit at the family dinner table.

"Scott, you are not in an ambulance. Slow down."

Food is one of the basic needs of life. When one has to eat fast to finish, that is a strong incentive.

One might ask, why don't they put a little refrigerator and plug for a hot plate or microwave in the ambulance? With technology today it shouldn't be too hard. Oh, wouldn't that be nice? Here's the reality:

Private ambulance companies are out to make a profit, at least a little bit. Public ambulances have to survive on as small a budget as possible. The ambulance bill is so high for a reason. Many people don't, can't, or won't pay. If all those who do are averaged with those who don't, the ambulance company makes about forty cents on the dollar. The company will cut the fat on equipment as much as the local regulatory agency will allow, but there's a limit. That leaves the employee. Turn the ambulance around for another call as quick as possible and tell them to bring their own food. The other fact is some numbskull would burn down the ambulance and sue the company for ruining their Panini.

Two days later James and I had a student, Raymond, riding with us. We were well into our shift and needing some dinner. James asked Dispatch if we could go out of service for some food.

"Are we clear for a Code 7 pickup at 16th and V?"

The dispatcher recognized where we were headed. A fantastic burrito place operated at 16th and Valencia. The answer however was, "Negative. We've got a call right around the corner I want you to handle. Code 2 for the leg injury, 16th and Albion, on 6-4-1."

James keyed the mike.

"Copy. 16th and Albion on 6-4-1. We're on it."

My stomach was about to rebel and I was getting irritable but we had accepted the call. James, relaxed and smiling, knew running a call would not impede our meal.

We drove over to the address, literally half a block away from our intended dinner stop. James turned to me and laid out the instructions.

"Raymond and I got this. Scott, I want the chicken burrito supreme with hot sauce. Make sure they use the red sauce. I don't want none of that wimpy green shit."

A twinge of conscience hit me. Should I leave my partner and go stand in line for our dinner? It didn't feel right. We should be focused on treating our patient. An hour wouldn't kill us. I needed to at least say something.

"Are you sure about this?"

"You're right. I'll go with the carne asada. That is some good shit. Same red sauce, though."

At this point we all stood around the patient, a homeless guy reclining against a chain link fence. He appeared alert, able to walk and carry on a conversation. James shooed me off to buy dinner while Raymond moved in to introduce himself.

I came out a few minutes later with a fine selection of burritos and chips. James and Raymond had our man in the back of the ambulance and were finishing up a discussion about the infection on his leg.

"Now, sir. You need to get that leg looked at," Raymond counseled.

James sat in the jump seat scribbling the routine stuff on the chart while Raymond did the dance to cover our butts because our patient was going to decide to go his own way in about five minutes.

"Thank you. I will. I have to go over to the hospital tomorrow anyway for my methadone."

"Well, all right. So long as you know it needs to be taken care of soon. Like, within the next day or two."

"Thank you, my friends."

"You're welcome. Sign the form."

James handed over the clipboard with the paper folded to present the signature line.

The patient limped out of the ambulance with Raymond's assist while James got on the radio.

"C-MED, eighty-eight's clear 16th and Albion on an advise/refuse. Can we pick up that Code 7 now?"

"You haven't gotten that yet? Yeah, you're clear. Out of service for thirty minutes on a Code 7 pickup."

Thirty minutes was all we needed.

CHAPTER 17

Oops, "Sorry."

James and I sat in the front of the ambulance, our little fishbowl, at Cal-Van, the corner of California and Van Ness. We hid in the back of a parking lot, tucked under a tree to cut down on the streetlights glaring through the windows, a solid concern at three in the morning.

James rolled the dial on the stereo while I ate more of my five-hour-old burrito. Whoever drove got the privilege of choosing the station and we switched driver and attendant every six hours. James made tonight's selection, "San Francisco Style," an interesting talk show with two hosts who spent the time reporting, interviewing, and discussing the events and issues of the Lesbian, Gay, Bisexual, Transgender, Queer, Intersex, and Asexual community—a community many areas of the country didn't care to recognize. Considered fringe elsewhere, the LGBTQIA had found an accepting home in San Francisco and a platform on this radio show to discuss ideas and provide information and support. I loved that aspect of San Francisco: Not getting heard in this city didn't mean you were an outcast, just a poorly organized minority. And the LGBTQIA in San Francisco were NOT poorly organized.

For me, growing up in white bread Midwestern suburbia, LGBTQIA was a new and amazing topic.

I learned how Johnny became Jane and that Max could decide whether to walk around as Maxine or Max because, being intersex, they had a choice. I learned sexual identity is quite a fluid concept and isn't a concrete aspect of our being.

"Eighty-eight."

Dispatch beckoned. I responded briskly, otherwise Richard got testy. "Eighty-eight. Cal-Van."

"Eighty-eight, we need you to head over to 1368 Jones, Apartment 6, for the med eval. Some guy says he's sick. Code 2 on 6-4-8."

"1368 Jones, number 6 on 6-4-8 for the sick. En route."

I finished scribbling the information on the log sheet. James dropped the shaft into drive and we slowly inched onto the street from our little hiding place.

We took off for an area on Nob Hill, a ritzy part of town, to meet a patient who showered recently and signaled a change in our clientele from the last few days. On the drive over I returned to finishing my burrito and learning about the issues of lesbians as they organized a charity auction to support an upcoming political issue.

In front of 1368 Jones, we poured ourselves out of the ambulance. I took a moment to stretch the kinks out of my back before walking to the side door and grabbing the jump kit. I never traveled without the jump kit. It held the BVM, the thing keeping me from doing mouth-to-mouth on people other than my wife.

I left the heart monitor and the oxygen bag. In San Francisco Dispatch, paramedics took the medical calls — the same folks I might be working with next week on the street. When they sent us out Code Two, a veteran paramedic already talked to the reporting party on the phone, asked a battery of the same questions I was about to ask, and had a firm idea I was walking in on something pretty minor.

With the jump kit digging a canyon in my shoulder, we headed off toward the elevator. Considering the neighborhood, we knew we'd find one and it would work.

Inside the building hung expensive chandeliers. The foyer had a bench to sit on and fresh, thick carpet. I could never afford it, but I sure enjoyed walking around.

We stepped into the spacious elevator. Well, in San Francisco terms. I wasn't going to be doing surgery there. However, I had room to stand far enough away from James that I couldn't evaluate his need for a breath mint, though he likely needed one. We exited the elevator to a posh hallway with two doors.

Ooh, two apartments per floor.

I prepared myself to experience décor only about three times out of my price range.

The door opened upon our knock and a well-dressed woman (remember, three in the morning) let us barely inside the foyer. Blocking further advancement into the apartment, she chortled, "Robert, it's time to go. The ambulance is here."

She strode to the nearby table, grabbed her purse and began to shrug on her coat.

This didn't work for me. I decided to reestablish the hierarchy right away.

"Good morning, ma'am. Whom are we here to see?"

"My husband. If you'll wait, he'll be here in a second and we can go to the hospital."

"Right. Well, there's an exam to do and some questions to ask. Is he this way?" I said, pointing down the hall to the main room of the apartment.

"Well, um, yes . . . ."

"Thank you."

Big smile and I turned to find Robert.

Not used to being questioned, she countered, "Um, excuse me."

James smoothly stepped in to redirect her attention.

"Good morning, ma'am. Will you show me your husband's medications? And I also have some questions for you," as he led her off to the kitchen.

I tell my paramedic students: When you arrive on scene, what the patient wants is about ninety percent irrelevant. This doesn't mean to be rude. It means the paramedic holds the most medical knowledge, should do a detailed exam and weigh the findings, and then decide what will and will not happen in light of those findings. In other words, the paramedic is in charge. Nothing happens without his or her permission and the flow of the call will progress at the rate set by the paramedic. If order isn't established in this fashion, someone else will attempt to establish it and the call won't go as efficiently.

Then there are those who need to know the world doesn't dance around their every whim.

I walked into the room and found Robert, I would guess, sitting on the sofa looking a little pale.

"Good morning. My name is Scott, what's your name?"

"Robert. Robert Jeffries."

In his sixties, he appeared generally healthy, only slightly overweight, well-kept, in slacks and a button-down shirt. The way they dressed in the middle of the night, the furnishings about the house, and how they carried themselves painted them to be long-time residents, well-to-do, conservative folks who would only call an ambulance for a true problem and as a last resort.

Mr. Jeffries glanced at me only briefly before refocusing on whatever mental turmoil held his full attention. Combining this action with his pale skin color, I agreed: He had an issue needing some quick investigation.

"What brings us here?"

"Well, I feel dizzy, and I want to throw up."

I opened the jump kit and pulled out the stethoscope and blood pressure cuff. Soon I had Mr. Jeffries' blood pressure at one hundred and thirty-four over seventy. His pulse proved strong and steady at one hundred and four, a little fast but anxiety might be in play. His skin was moist, another valid sign, or an increasing tally for anxiety.

Most signs and symptoms had such a hurdle: They all listed correctly from several medical complaints. Only when added up and compared to the story from the patient did I hope to piece together a hint of a cause.

"Sir, how long has your stomach been bothering you?"

While he answered I also evaluated his speech patterns and looked for drooping in his face or trouble moving his arms or legs as signs of a stroke.

"It started tonight. About three hours ago."

"And what were you doing when it started?"

"I was about to go to bed. I have been sitting here hoping it would go away, but it hasn't."

He answered clearly and quickly. His brain seemed to be working and he was getting enough oxygen to understand my question and formulate an appropriate answer.

"You say it's been going on for about three hours?"

He didn't answer right away. His eyes appeared to glaze over but then refocused.

That was weird. I asked the question again.

"So, this has been going on for about three hours?"

His eyes glazed over, just for a second.

"Sir, did you just feel any different? Did your vision change at all?"

"Huh? It was that nauseous thing again."

I got a funny twinge in my own stomach. Something bad was happening. I couldn't figure it out yet, but I sensed the need to get moving, find out more things, and start developing an exit plan.

"Hey James," I said.

"Yeah?" James' voice filtered back to me.

"Can you bring up the stair chair? Something's happening here and I would like to move downstairs."

"Sure. I'll be right back."

And James sauntered out of the room.

I had a few minutes to wait.

I kept a hold on Mr. Jeffries' wrist. A steady, strong pulse pressed against my fingers. I asked him more questions.

"Did you get a little dizzy about a minute ago?"

"Yeah, a little woozy. That's been happening all night."

An idea what I might be seeing began to formulate. He might be passing out for the shortest amount of time. But what was the cause? Volume loss or dilation of the vessels wouldn't be temporary and he'd be down and on his back.

This might be a heart rhythm irregularity. I hadn't caught one yet, but I also had not held his pulse for a long time. If his heart was throwing out enough irregular beats, his blood output would drop, disrupting the flow to the brain. If the brain gets a disruption for any amount of time, it becomes cranky and goes on strike.

Back to my questions. "Sir, when you're dizzy, does your vision change? Does your eyesight go gray or black?"

"I don't seem to notice anything. My eyes haven't been the same for years, you know. I lost my reading glasses a couple of weeks ago. They really do the job for me."

Mrs. Jeffries, freed when James left the house, wandered back to find us.

"Excuse me. It's time to go to the hospital. Our physician has been notified and will be waiting for us at California Pacific Medical Center. We've delayed this long enough."

I had no intention of getting into a pissing match with this lady even though I had a firm notion their physician was not crawling from under the covers, pulling on pants, and kissing the spouse. They would be waiting until the awake and working emergency room doc called and gave a complete and informed report before deciding to make the drive in.

"Yes, ma'am." I turned to face Mrs. Jeffries while still keeping a hand on Robert's wrist. "My partner left to retrieve a chair for your husband. After completing my exam there are reasons I do not want Mr. Jeffries walking downstairs."

"Well, he's been poorly all night, but if we left when you got here, we would be at the hospital by now."

"Yes, ma'am. That would be true . . . if he made it down the stairs without passing out and hitting his head, causing further injury."

"Oh, you're just being melodramatic. Our doctor, Dr. Richard Grestorian, the best in the City, gave Robert a clean bill of health last week. His stomach is bothering him. I only called you because I prefer not to drive at night."

This was turning into the pissing match I didn't want.

"Yes ma'am." *You old biddy.*

Mrs. Jeffries glared at me.

There. Was that a missed beat or did my hand slip?

I looked at his eyes. He was coming back from another short trip of unconsciousness.

Damn. Where was James with the stair chair? I wanted to move this guy downstairs and get him hooked up to the heart monitor. He had problems I needed to see with my own eyes.

The Ambulance Gods heard my plea because James returned. He flipped open the stair chair and I filled him in on my findings so far.

"I think he's having arrhythmias and they're causing syncope. Let's get him downstairs."

We both worked swiftly to load Mr. Jeffries onto the chair. I tipped him back and we rolled off to the elevator, gathering Mrs. Jeffries as we headed to the front door.

I smiled at her as we passed, intending to mean one of several things, whichever way she decided. One, a pleasant smile to build confidence that Mr. Jeffries was being well-cared for. Two, a peace offering. Or three, a smug grin to let her know, yes, the "staff" usurped her and we were now following my plan. Didn't matter to me which one she picked. By her not looking at me and the way she held her gaze straight ahead, I guessed she went with option three. We all piled into the elevator, James, our patient, his wife, and me with my bag creating a tight squeeze as I kept a hold on Mr. Jeffries' pulse at his wrist.

It happened again. He glazed over and I definitely felt a space in the beats of his pulse.

"There," I said to James. "That's the third time he's glazed over since we've been here."

Then I remembered I was also talking in front of Mrs. Jeffries and she deserved a détente between us. I didn't need two patients.

"Ma'am, what I'm seeing is your husband seems to blank out for a few seconds. We're going down to the ambulance to check a few things out after which we'll depart for the hospital as soon as we can."

I followed that up with a genuine, caring smile meant to put her at ease over her husband's condition. Didn't work. I think she was still pissed at me. *Whatever.*

The elevator doors opened with the ambulance directly out front. I didn't want to slow things down so I directed Mrs. Jeffries as we rolled through the lobby.

"Ma'am, can you just hop in the front and put your seatbelt on? We'll be leaving in a few minutes. Like I said, we're going to check some things and then we'll get rolling."

I followed up with a "Thank you."

James and I rolled Mr. Jeffries to the rear of the ambulance. I opened the doors and we hefted him inside. Done properly, lifting someone is only marginally bad on my back. Multiply by thirty to forty years and I should only be crippled a little.

I directed Robert to slide over to the gurney after which James took the stair chair out and refolded it to its holder on the side door.

I grabbed the electrode wires out of the pocket of the heart monitor to see the answers that were a little pressing. The three stickers were already applied and I slapped one on his right upper chest, one to his left upper chest and the third on his left belly. I flipped on the monitor and the green light blipped across the screen in a pattern spelling healthy.

Well, that was kind of what I expected to find. I felt a normal pulse rate most of the time. I wanted to snag a picture of the other stuff.

James climbed back inside the ambulance and pulled out a nasal cannula. Some oxygen in the nose ought to boost our patient's condition. His lungs were working fine, but his brain kept checking out and was obviously unhappy at some points. A little extra help wouldn't hurt. James strapped the tubing over his ears. My eyes never left the heart monitor.

There! My question was answered.

Oh, shit!

The monitor showing Mr. Jeffries' heart rhythm went from blipping merrily and healthily along to an absolute straight line, asystole. His eyes fluttered and glazed over. The screen was one completely straight line, no rhythm at all, for about seven seconds and then the beats came back. Mr. Jeffries regained focus as he said, "Yep, there was that dizziness again."

Damn! I'll say.

"James, can you start the ignition for some light in here?"

We now had a laundry list of things to worry about and I did not want to add a dead ambulance battery.

James reached through and cranked the engine to life.

Thank God that was cooperative.

James retook his seat and began stripping out an IV line while I ripped open a pack of pacer pads. These were an improvement over the gel we used to use that, if it ran together on the patient's chest, would make a blue arc and burn the skin.

With the pads we could also pace the patient, applying smaller jolts of electricity to help slow heart rates.

Now that I knew Mr. Jeffries' problem, I realized he was lucky to have any rhythm whatsoever show up on the monitor and the quicker I got the pads on, the better. At any moment the next heartbeat might not happen and I'd be doing chest compressions. On the other hand, scaring the man by showing my fears might do the job, too. Urgency without acting like it was in order.

"Mr. Jeffries, I need you to remove your shirt, please."

I helped him with the buttons and kept explaining what I was about to do, using my calming but professional voice.

"I need to put some large sticky pads on your chest and back. Your dizziness is caused by your heart not acting normally. If it does this too much, frankly, it could kill you." I added a brief smile to try and lighten the topic. "With these pads, I'll be able to keep that from happening."

Mr. Jeffries responded to my assessment.

"Wow, um, by all means, let's put those pads on."

"Thank you, Sir."

With his shirt removed, I peeled the eight-inch by eight-inch pad off its plastic storage panel.

"Can you lean forward, sir? This pad goes on your back."

I stuck the pad firmly to the left side of his back, below the shoulder blade.

"Thank you. Lean back. The next one goes on your chest."

The second pad I placed over his left breast and plugged them both into the heart monitor.

Now with the pacer pads on, all we needed to do in case Mr. Jeffries decided to stay in his slow (zero) heart rate was flip a dial and we caught him as he fell, so to speak. Currently, he had a pulse. His blood pressure was actually quite normal. I wanted to keep that in mind. It helped me relax. Not everything was in the shitter yet. Only for short periods. We still had room to work.

Next I needed an intravenous line. Electricity was a nice medication and it could be applied rapidly, but it was also rather abrupt and I've had at least one patient say, "Oh, don't do that again," as I approached them the second time with the paddles.

With an IV line, I could give Mr. Jeffries some Valium for relaxation in case I had to zap him. Valium also has an amnesic effect, reducing his memory of the whole thing. The thought of being zapped with something like a baseball bat to the chest made me think amnesia would be ideal. And finally, with an IV, in case Mr. Jeffries continued to throw me curve balls, I could keep up with him using the cabinet full of medications stored six inches from his right shoulder.

James finished prepping the line and laying out the items needed to start the IV.

The voice of Mrs. Jeffries warbled from up front.

"Um, excuse me. Can we go to the hospital now?"

Damn it! I thought we had worked out who was in charge. Who did she think she called? A cab?

This was an ambulance and essentially an extension of the emergency department. I didn't need an extra level of stress. Old Bob, here, threatened to check out to higher grounds and my job entailed making sure he didn't find his ticket for transit.

Mrs. Jeffries might be used to having her way but this was my ambulance. Tomorrow she could swill champagne for breakfast, raise her pinky during tea time, and hobnob with the rest of the conservatives over dinner. Right now I had more pressing issues and following her flow chart was not on my list.

"I'm sorry, ma'am. Your husband's very sick. We've got a lot to do back here, for the moment. We'll start moving as soon as I get this IV."

I wrapped the tourniquet, swabbed Mr. Jeffries' arm clean, and stuck him with the catheter. I taped down my handiwork and a voice warbled from the front again.

"Um, excuse me."

"Yes, ma'am?" I tried not to, but my voice sounded a little strained.

She continued.

"Must we listen to this?"

For a second I was confused.

Oops, Sorry. "San Francisco Style."

We left the radio on and Mrs. Jeffries found herself, at that moment, being educated about the needs of the transgender in our fair city. She was perhaps unaware they had needs. She most probably did not spend a lot of her day even acknowledging this sort of community. We were broadening Mrs. Jeffries' world. A lot.

"I'm sorry, ma'am."

I leaned forward and punched off the radio. Inside I giggled.

James got out and strode to the front to drive us to the hospital. Everything was going to be all right. We now had Mr. Jeffries covered with an IV and pacer pads, if he needed them. He was on the way to get a pacemaker put in because he couldn't tolerate many more episodes of the games his heart was playing.

During the quiet drive toward the hospital I overheard Mrs. Jeffries speaking to James.

"I don't find it appropriate having such things on the radio and my husband is in the back."

James replied, showing his best.

"I apologize, ma'am. We were listening to the show earlier and the radio was on when we turned off the engine. We're taking good care of your husband. His heart is in a precarious spot and I am very glad you called us to give him the care we can provide. We'll be at the hospital very shortly and I'll help you out as the step down can be a bit long."

"Thank you, young man."

As for the Lesbian, Gay, Bisexual, Transgender, and Queer community? Maybe they had a new benefactor in Mrs. Jeffries.

Probably not.

CHAPTER 18

Bad Weed

"Eighty-eight, copy Code 2."

I keyed the mike clipped to my shoulder. "Eighty-eight. Division and South Van."

"Eighty-eight, we've got one for you. 352 11th Street, Code 2, for the eval."

Richard continued the readout and I scribbled the information on the run sheet, repeating it back, per protocol.

James, driving for his half of the shift, took a quick glance out his window before executing a U-turn in the intersection to point us in the right direction. With a grin on his face he said, "Heh, heh. This one's definitely yours."

"Why? What's at 352 11th?"

My suspicions always rose when James smiled.

"Oh, you'll see. They're gonna fuckin' *love* you."

"Whatever. Just drive."

352 11th Street was a bar. Over the doorway hung a square, white sign with simple black letters declaring, "SF Durango."

James double-parked, blocking the lane of traffic, and we met on the sidewalk. I had the jump kit, he carried the clipboard. With an exaggerated flourish and a courteous "after you," James waved me toward the door and past the lavish décor of plywood painted black.

Instantly assaulted by a heavy bass rhythm, I walked into an open room filled to the brim with the bar's patrons who added to the cacophony of sound.

I peered over the crowd to the far end of the room anchored by a stage and its stupendously large speakers, looking for a clue where my patient might be. I observed during my scan the preponderance of men. Upon even further analysis, I saw the bar was jam-packed with only men and all wearing leather. I had never seen so many men and dead cow in one room at one time. I was in the biggest leather bar on the West Coast. Oh, my. And me from Ohio.

A man stepped in front of me, blocking my path. I tensed, ready to jump in any direction. He made no further move toward me. In fact, his eyes said he was bored. He motioned for us to follow and dove into the crowd of leather-clad men.

I noted, as we bumped our way past, the dress code covered a limited array of outfits. The full leather coat and leather pants ensemble seemed popular. Others displayed the coat, jeans and chaps collection after which we had the leather vest over a bare chest. Some midriffs were not flattering. Next, we arrived at the vest-and-chaps-only crowd. Chaps, being so constructed, tend to leave areas open to the wind. To compensate, the wearer encased his vital parts in a leather thong. A few had forgotten their thong.

I kept my head down, trying not to stare at the flagrant displays — I didn't want any trouble, I didn't want any dates — while we followed our fully-clothed guide spearheading a meager path through the herd to eventually move up on stage, along with its speakers and the source of the penetrating bass.

From this vantage point I had an expansive overview of the crowd. I put the number at five hundred guys in this one room and quite an impressive sight: All men and all wearing black leather.

One man was shorter than the rest. His head rose about as tall as another man's belt. Actually, no . . . .

Oh, God.

We stepped off the stage on the other side to arrive at my patient, a fresh-faced white boy dressed in the seemingly prerequisite leather. He, however, had a more conservative fashion sense and wore his outerwear over some innerwear.

I shouted over the bass and the sheer number of men.

"Hey. What's going on tonight?"

He rocked band and forth on a step, arms wrapping his knees, while his eyes darted around the room.

"I don't feel good. I think I'm freaking out."

"Why? What did you do?" I took his wrist to grab a ballpark count on his pulse. It was a little fast.

"I don't know. I just don't feel right."

"What do you mean by not feeling right?"

"Sort of . . . I don't know. Not right."

Irritation flowed up my neck. I found hollering over the noise of a stuffed bar and trying to catch feeble utterances annoying. This guy didn't appear to be in impressive distress but his answers failed to move this whole thing forward.

A man on the step behind spoke up. At first, he appeared to be on top of the boy, but no, he in fact sat like a second skin, draped over and providing soft strokes. Despite the glue-like presentation, the man gave the answer I sought.

"He's new around here. Smoked his first weed tonight."

A wash of relief settled over me. My patient wasn't going to die in the next five minutes. He still had two legs and, as long as they were attached, it was time to walk.

I gave a tug on my patient's wrist.

"Let's go outside and talk about this."

"Can I come?" Glue Guy had unstuck himself enough to let the boy stand, but not much more.

"Sure."

To keep the flow going.

Our little posse traveled back through the herd, arriving outside to a starry, and quieter, night.

In the ambulance we put Reefer Boy on the gurney, prompting his friend, Mr. Sticky, to grab the seat behind his head. I sat on the bench to begin my interview while James started taking vital signs.

"My name's Scott. What's yours?"

"Jason Barnes."

151

I scribbled out the personal information as he fed it to me. Time to rehash the story.

"So, what's going on tonight?"

"I don't know. I just feel weird."

Jason rocked on the gurney, holding himself in a hug.

'Feeling weird' wouldn't cut it. I needed something to put on the chart explaining why we had met and, if we were going to the hospital, to tell the doctor. Basically, I required more adjectives. I opted for the short, simple approach.

"Your friend here tells me you smoked some marijuana tonight. Is that true?"

"Well, um . . ."

"Listen. I'm not the cops. I'm not going to tell the cops. My interest is to hear the whole story, figure out if something's going to really hurt you, and decide where to go from there. So, did you do any weed?"

"Um, yes," he squeaked and buried his face as if he had told the Pope he didn't like the communion bread.

Oh God. I sat back in frustration. This was like trying to interview Bashful, the Dwarf, about his erections.

I shifted my gaze from the patient up to his friend who knew something earlier. I didn't have to go far. While perched on the edge of the seat, he stroked Jason's hair.

"The weed. How was the source? Could it have been cut with anything?"

"No, man. It was clean. I've been toking up all night."

Well, this guy appeared to be handling his smoke all right. He talked straight and his eyes weren't doing interesting circles.

James turned, pulled the leads from the heart monitor and stuck them on Jason's chest.

When the monitor screen lit up, our boy's heart clicked along at about 130 beats per minute. Too fast for sitting still.

"Hey Jason, did you do any drugs tonight?"

"No. Why? What's going on?"

Jason kept scanning the ambulance and wringing his hands. I couldn't decide whether he was the nervous type and not enjoying his first date with Mary Jane or if he had mixed and matched. Hell, maybe someone had slipped him something. One thing for certain, if I didn't calm this guy down in about ten minutes, heart rate below one hundred, we were off to the hospital.

"Well, Jason. Your heart's going a little fast for what we're all doing here. Any ideas?"

Jason's eyes went wide and he sat up straight, grabbing the handrails. "What? What do you mean?"

"What I mean is your heart is going at about 130 beats a minute. For me to get my heart that fast, I would have to go for a jog. You're doing it sitting still. Did you do anything besides the weed?"

He relaxed his grip but he was still skittish. "No. I just don't feel good. I don't know anything."

I looked at his eyes. People say they are the window to the soul. He was telling the truth. I felt pretty sure this was nerves, but I have to continually remind myself where I reside in the medical hierarchy – right near the bottom, to where "things" roll after coming downhill. We were going to the doctor.

"We'll take you in. Which hospital do you want to go to?"

"Never been to one."

"Davies is the closest. Sound okay to you?" Jason nodded and curled on the gurney while his friend continued to stroke his hair and coo soft encouragements.

"All right. Davies it is."

To James I said, "Let's go."

James turned and stepped to go out, but stopped.

"Where do you want him?"

Normally, friends or relatives didn't ride in the back. It's a security thing. Sometimes I let it slide. I shouldn't, but I get vibes off people. These two seemed okay. Besides, they could keep each other company — and I didn't have a pry bar.

"He can stay." To the friend, "Buckle your seat belt."

"Okay," said the man. He fumbled around, located the belt under the seat, buckled up, and returned to caressing.

It was a short ride to the hospital with most of my time spent writing the chart and filling in the story with a few more answered questions. I wanted to finish so we could drop this guy and be gone, maybe grab a coffee, before dispatch thought about giving us another call.

My keeping busy didn't bother the boys. They tested the limits of the belts trying to touch as much as possible. I felt voyeuristic over the heated action two feet beyond my boots. Young love. How sweet.

We pulled into the ambulance parking. Once inside, I waited to begin my report until the nurse looked ready. "Looking ready" consisted of lifting her pen from the chart and gazing up. Gail had seen way too much to be impressed.

"We've got a twenty-two-year-old male who seems to have smoked his first weed tonight which isn't sitting too well with him. He's a little tachy, doing 130, and he says he doesn't feel well. He says he's got no chest pain and no abdominal pain, just that he doesn't feel well."

Gail stopped me with a slightly raised hand. She pointed and James escorted the patient, with his friend, to the closest treatment room. She allowed a slight nod for me to continue.

"He was a little jumpy for the ride in. He says he hasn't done any other drugs beyond a mixed drink and his friend says the marijuana came from a solid source, so it shouldn't be cut with anything interesting."

Gail started to look bored so I quickly finished my report. "He says he's got no pertinent medical history, takes no meds, and has no allergies."

With a voice matching her face she said, "Thanks. I'll see to him in a minute." She went back to writing on the chart in her hand.

I always tried to leave with a little levity. "For the next one I'll bring you something with more teeth."

Gail threw me a weak smile without stopping her pen. "Don't bother. This will do. I don't need the headache."

I glanced at the board showing the patient census. She had a full house.

"Sorry. I'll go easy on you the rest of the night."

This time she offered me a glint and a smile.

"No, you won't. You love us too much."

"You're right."

I stepped off to finish my chart.

A few minutes later I slid the completed chart into the rack for my patient's bed. I turned and walked into Jason's room. I liked to make a habit, at least for the patients who didn't piss me off, to stop in and say goodbye.

Jason sat on the gurney; his friend was in his usual spot attempting to split atoms between them.

I smiled.

"All right, Jason. You take care. Don't do any more marijuana. It doesn't seem to sit too well with you."

"Thank you. I appreciate you guys taking care of me."

"You're welcome."

I turned to leave the room. The friend spoke up as I reached the door.

"Excuse me. Can two people fit on these gurneys?"

I didn't even want to visualize how far that would go.

"No. Trade phone numbers and make a date."

CHAPTER 19

Christmas With The Eberharts

Happy Holidays to all. Another year is coming to a
close. The family is intact, more of us speak in full sentences
and fewer of us drool on a regular basis. Almost all
mastered silverware, while coloring between the lines is still
a challenge for many. We survived our continued hectic
schedules and all, in our own little ways, grew.

We, The Adults (smirk)

Many changes occurred this year. The San Francisco Fire
Department moved everyone to twenty-four-hour shifts
with me now working a simple schedule of every third day
with five days off every third week. I spend my work days
running lots of calls and learning which end of the fire hose
to use. Two years ago, I would have said, "Firefighter? Nah,
not something I'll probably ever do." Now, I wear turnout
pants, red suspenders, a coat which is too hot and heavy in
the summer, I slide down a pole while half asleep and
wonder what the heck I'm supposed to do at a fire. The
good changes are, I eat meals using silverware without a
steering wheel in my gut and sleep in a real bed instead of
the gurney in the back of the ambulance.

Camille continues to work in the E.D. and goes to
school, taking classes to certify as a Legal Nurse Consultant.
Once she gets going, her schedule will free up a little more.
She'll still work at the hospital to keep current, fresh, and
varied. These are long-range plans. Until then, it is business
as usual with the calendar reigning supreme in the
household.

The Getting-Older One

Justine is now ten, taller and changing. One can speak in
deep philosophical tones and she responds with "the look."
One can say, "Justine, are you getting ready for school?"
Half an hour later she's actually done. She is caring about
her clothes and shows taste. She does hair things which are
quite impressive and we are still able to send her out the
door.

Them

These are the reasons we continue to emphatically state
we will create no more children. We love them dearly but,
as I will demonstrate, trying to keep up with more than
these would kill us. Kylene smashed her first birthday cake
this year and does things when she damn well pleases.
Smiling and laughing? Not until she could walk. She was
headed for a future in Las Vegas at the poker tables until
she decided to smile. We planned a camping trip for a few
months after we thought she would be walking. Someone
told Kylene, I'm sure. We spent three days hunched over as
Kylene would not walk anywhere without a hand to hold.
She screamed her way over hill and dale in the backpack
attached to Daddums. We went with another family. Their
child said to Scott, halfway up some Everest-like mountain,
   "Doesn't that screaming bother you?"
   Ah, children.
   Elise, headed toward that third birthday, added her fun
to this communing with nature. She threw up at three a.m.
the first night. Picture us draping an encrusted child over a
picnic bench at "0" dark thirty. The sun rose and so did
Kylene, which awoke Elise howling.
   The man in the tent next door yelled, "Shut up!"
   Lesson in futility # 1: Telling a two-and-a-half-year-old
to stop crying and go back to sleep. We will not be camping
again until the children are older.

After the camping experience, Kylene decided to walk and is having a blast. She laughs and smiles crossing the room. She, however, has not yet talked. Nary a word. We know she understands as we can say,

"Go back and pick that up and put it in the garbage."

And she will. Someday she'll talk, we hold no worries because . . .

. . . Elise. I saw a sweatshirt. It said, "I've started talking and I can't shut up." She's all legs and thin and Scott's brother doesn't help when he spends the weekend teaching her, "Elise, repeat after me, 'I have no butt. '" It's true, but it doesn't help.

Elise likes to put things together. She does well at puzzles and she likes to color and paint. Since September she's been going to preschool twice a week. She does other things, mostly when Scott's home alone with the small ones, like crayons and walls, chalk and carpet, lipstick and face (got a picture of that one). The crème de la crème occurred a short time ago.

An Elise Moment

It began simply enough, as most disasters do. I was on the phone setting up an appointment.

Elise bounced over to me and said with stress in her voice, "I have to go potty."

She's been potty trained for about two months now but I still ask, "Do you need help?"

She responded with her newest independence.

"No."

And off she went to the bathroom.

At that moment the forces of evil converged on my house, quietly moving inside to cause several things to happen at once. My first hint was the sound of running water. This and almost-three-year-olds are not a safe mixture, especially when spontaneously created. But, I thought the best of my little gem as she solidified her bathroom technique.

"Ah, she's washing her hands."

This is something which should be monitored but, for the moment, all the water funneled down the sink.

The unsettled howl of Elise alerted me to the undeniable presence of a problem. The pitch of her trumpeting suggested a quick investigation. I rounded the corner to find her sitting on the rug with her pants at her ankles. This was not the problem.

The forces of evil deftly accomplished two things at once. Elise plugged the toilet. It is a low-flow toilet, so this happens a lot. Not a big issue. When Elise flushed the toilet, the flapper inside the tank stuck, thus allowing the toilet to gleefully do its job of refilling the bowl—forever. Much like Hawaii's Mauna Kea pouring lava on the terrified inhabitants of the village below, the toilet flowed from all exits down the bowl and onto the floor.

Elise resembled a damp little island on the soaked rug with the floor 1/4" deep in rushing water. There existed a good side to this event. Most of the water did not flow out of the bathroom and to the hardwood to be soaked up by an entirely too expensive rug. Most of the water flowed briskly across the floor and dove like Niagara's point of no return down the heater vent to points unknown. My first thought seemed surprisingly calm.

"Hmm, I wonder where that goes in regards to water."

My mission was now clear.

1. End the phone call.

"Beth, gotta go. My daughter flooded the bathroom."

2. Stop the overflowing toilet while not breaking the lid or any objects in the bathroom (to include the child).

3. Extract Elise from her watery torture of a damp butt.

4. Begin the process of cleaning up the mess before things soaked through and truly damaged something.

During this initial attack and rectification, Kylene The Curious walked serenely into the bathroom, surveyed the event up close, observed as Elise was airlifted over her into the hallway, and got her socks supremely wet.

Happy Holidays.

Love, the Eberharts

CHAPTER 20

Three A.M.

Three in the morning. San Francisco. In the ambulance at Union Square. I finished drooling on my right cheek and that made me happy. I liked tonight's little nap. The stereo, turned low for company, softly filled the space. The ambulance was warm, almost cozy. Mickey's hands declared I had been asleep ten minutes and we'd been sitting here for twenty-five: A veritable vacation.

Outside, the garbage truck motored its way around the Square in jerky stops and the hiss of compressed air. The men spun the cans across Post. Working in pairs, they traded the empties for full ones and skidded them to the truck in a twirling dance of plastic blue.

By three a.m. the night life electricity is pulled at the plug. Last Call was an hour ago and the social drunkards were either home or collected by one of the city's services. Tonight we successfully avoided that type. I hated battling the immature drunks and cleaning up the mess they left on my floor.

What didn't go away were the Night People. We drove by and saw men and women standing on the corners, leaning up on the buildings, talking in small groups. What is talked about at three in the morning?

"Nice weather we're having, although a little dark."

Welcome to San Francisco, home of the cable cars — the only moving National Historic Monument, the Giants, the Niners, and eight hundred fifty thousand people stuffed into forty-nine square miles. The City swelled to over 1 million during the day with the commuters and tourists, but I wouldn't know. James and I lived on the night shift . . . weekends.

James lay stretched out on the gurney, snoring a lot. I used to go in back to nap. I would spread a sheet over the bench to hide what I cleaned but might have missed, hang the radio on a hook, and let the microphone dangle by my ear. A blanket became my pillow and I covered up with my coat. Just like home. But I didn't do that anymore. I might miss a call.

Missing a call was not hard. We received no pages, no alerting tones or other, "It's for you" niceties. We only had the portable radio and the dispatcher calling our ambulance number. Last week the paramedic supervisor opened the back door and woke us both up. He advised us Dispatch tried to reach us for twenty-three minutes and the next time we "went to the bathroom at the hospital," one of us should stay outside in case we were in a radio dead zone.

"Eighty-eight."

A disembodied voice dropped out of the speaker clipped on my shoulder. Three things must happen nearly simultaneously. I had to grab the clipboard lying on the floor, then ready a pen. Thirdly, I had to answer back in less than 3.7 seconds. Any longer and Richard got testy. A pissed-off dispatcher could lock me out from any other part of the City my entire career.

I responded briskly with my unit number and location using my best 'awake' voice.

"Eighty-eight. Square."

Dispatchers knew medics dozed off or even gargled, brushed, and bedded down for the night. To broadcast with the 'you just woke me up' voice was poor form.

Richard droned into my shoulder. "Eighty-eight. Code 2 for the eight-oh-one. 342 Eddy, apartment 412, on 3-5-4."

I pressed the mic key. "Eighty-eight copies. 342 Eddy on 3-5-4."

I scribbled the readout on the log sheet following the boxes intended for each bit of information. An 801 was cop talk for suicide attempt. We still used their radio code because we didn't want to broadcast some suicidal guy lived on Eddy Street. Of course, in the Tenderloin, he had plenty of company.

Time to wake Sleeping Beauty.

"Hey, we got a Code 2. Suicide attempt."

"Shit," James mumbled and mixed in a groan.

I answered his rhetorical complaints.

"I don't request them. I just write them down. Slide your ass up here. Your turn to drive."

"I'm coming."

The rest became lost in bumps, groans, profanities, and the back door opening and slamming. The driver's door opened and James crawled into the seat.

With half-peeled eyes and a red sleep mark on his left cheek, he asked, "What are you looking at, you shit?"

Working with James was interesting. Crass and vulgar, his sense of humor bordered on insanity. His saving grace for keeping his job involved being polite when necessary and he was actually a damned good medic. He was fast and right about the medicine. A bad combo would be fast and wrong. I hated the idea of spending the shift babysitting my partner so he didn't kill somebody and get me fired in the process.

"What I'm looking at," I began, "is a guy who looks like hell and whose hair resembles a terrible mousse accident. Your eyes are bloodshot, your teeth have leftover green shit in them from a scrumptious burrito, of which half is still stuffed behind the seat, and you are about to go serve the sick and injured."

"Yeah, don't you fuckin' love it?" His grin widened to reveal more dinner refuse as he turned the key and forced the engine to life, barely. "Where to?"

"342 Eddy."

James dropped the lever into drive and jerked the ambulance away from the curb. Working with DPH for four years, he couldn't, or wouldn't, move off the night shift. He was a medic for eight years and on ambulances for "too fucking long," in his words.

He was honestly full of hot air. He, like the rest of us in the business, would have dried up and blown away without this job. Punching the ticket and sharpening pencils didn't make sense. He needed his nightly dose of adrenaline. Without it, he might turn cranky.

James drove draped over the wheel, avoiding cars and changing lanes by leaning. I had one foot up on the fake carpeted dash trying to avoid waking up completely.

We coasted under the streetlights to see someone who said he was going to kill himself. A successful attempt and the call would have been a Code 3, lights and siren, with an attached engine company from the Fire Department. No, this guy was making a statement and wanted the world to hear his plea. We were elected as the world's representatives.

We drifted away from Union Square and headed into the Tenderloin, the Loin for anybody who lived here. This part of town has been getting the shit end of the stick since way back. Supposedly, that was even how the name came about. The story, among others which may or may not be true, said a cop would transfer here and join the rest of the force shaking down the residents so he could afford to buy his family the better cut of meat, the tenderloin. That was one of the stories, anyway. Whichever, the locals still swam upstream trying to make the neighborhood more conducive to normal life.

We drifted through the streets until we pulled up half a block short. The one-way street went to the right, but we needed to turn left to reach the 300 block. James flipped on the emergency lights, turned left and split the meager three a.m. traffic headlights while I counted down the last addresses to 342 Eddy. After finding a section of open curb and shutting off the engine, James stared out the windshield and sighed deeply.

"All right. Let's go."

James got the clipboard and I grabbed the medical bag out of the side door. I used more of a lift to start the motion and followed the momentum as it swung out of the ambulance. The damn thing seemed heavier as the shift went on.

James and I met in the middle of the sidewalk and I glanced up at the building, a lovely example of Neo-something architecture. A solid structure of brick and stone, adorned with bars on the windows and a black security gate, she withstood all the City had forgotten. The fire escape lay tucked into its holder over the cracked and stained sidewalk where an odd paper scrap skittered toward the gutter. Someone didn't want it and that is what you did with things you didn't want, put them on the street.

A guy slept in the doorway next door. A quick visual suggested he was alive. Not because he could be seen breathing. He lay burrowed under who knows how many layers of coats and sweaters. His face was the right color, not blue, or death-violet. He was curled against the building and not splayed out. He showed a sense of purpose — to keep warm and unbothered. And he deserved at least that.

He slept with the look of someone never far from some anxiety. Tomorrow began another scramble to stay alive, to find more food in an unpicked trash can and drink a little relief from a bottle he scrounged. For now, he slept. At least we didn't have two patients.

James stepped toward the security gate and rang the buzzer for the night manager.

I stood near the ambulance.

"Isn't this the part where we're supposed to wait for the cops? You know, suicidal, couldn't care less about taking us with him?"

The gate released. James swung the grated metal door open and stepped inside.

"Yeah."

And he plodded off to find the stairs or, hopefully, an elevator.

I caught the gate as it closed.

As a first impression, the ground-floor lobby created a persona of dingy. Wallpaper someone thought a good idea at some time was now faded and peeled and scarcely showed its yellow velveteen flower design. In all fairness, the scenery was hard to truly appreciate in the light of the single bulb hanging by a cord. The carpet was dark colored. Intentionally? I hefted the bag and trudged through the lobby, shelving that question for another day. To the left sat the night manager in a caged office. The glow of a TV filled his space. I figured keeping track of the comings and goings of the place was his job, so I let him know our destination.

"Apartment 412."

He didn't move, presenting himself one notch above corpse and half that distance to caring.

James stood in front of the elevator until the car clattered to a stop and he forced the gate open. I squeezed past into the double telephone-booth-size room and put the bag on my feet. Stand any other way and the gate wouldn't close. It was cozy.

James pushed the "4" button. We started with a jolt and crawled up the inside of the bare shaft. The walls slid past and the doors of each floor lazily came down from the ceiling. I imagined attempting to open a passing door. That, however, would have been stupid because I would have gotten my hand stuck in the cage as the elevator rose, continuing its fight for the assigned floor.

"You know," James began to expound. "You gotta love these old things." He scanned our little rising box.

"They've been getting the job done for probably hundreds of years and now we have the added spice of possibly plummeting to the basement instead."

He smiled broadly at his observation.

I looked at my partner.

"You should clean that shit out of your teeth."

The elevator clanked to a stop at a door marked "4." James pulled the gate to the side. I pushed the door open and stepped into a long narrow version of the lobby with the bulbs, carpet, and sick wallpaper.

"What was the number?" I said over my shoulder as I began to locate rooms.

The clank of the clipboard let me know James heard me. His answer sounded tired.

"412."

The clunk of our heavy boots filling the hallway were now accompanied by the sucking sounds of James doing dental hygiene.

"James, how do you keep the women off you?"

"It's a gift."

"Uh huh. Here we go." I counted down the last few doors after finding the evens on the left side.

I stopped in front of a brown door which hadn't seen fresh paint since the dawn of time, and that would have been the fifth coat. On a flat portion at eye level, the numbers 412 were scrawled with black marking pen. We took up positions flanking the door with me on the far side. While leaning against the lovely wallpaper rather than standing straight, I noticed the underlying odors of the hallway had some prominent winners. Eau de cigarettes, urine, and general filth struck hard, forever trapped in the wallpaper and carpet.

When James and I first started working together, I made the mistake of standing in front of the door to knock. James knocked me silly as he pushed me off to the side.

"You dumb shit. They shoot through the door when you knock. If you want your guts, stand to the side."

Now, I leaned against the paper-thin wall. I had to stand somewhere.

I reached across and knocked firmly. Cannon volleys in the silence of the hallway.

"Ambulance."

Another cannon shot bounded toward the elevator.

The silence overtook quickly.

A meek voice came through the door.

"It's open."

My opening the door allowed the person inside to set up the timing for whatever ambush he planned. If I waited for him we would be here all night. I reached for the doorknob, twisted, and threw the door open.

Starting with a cheery opener always seemed polite.

"Good evening, Sir."

The 'Sir' in reference sat on the bed to the right side of the single room/oversized closet where he presumably lived. The rest of the room swelled with a sink containing various science projects in full bloom; shelves brimming with clothes; towels and dark masses of objects I cared not to decipher at this hour; stacked pots and pans I assumed were used on the hot plate stored atop the tiny refrigerator sitting on the little wooden chair; nudie magazines, all titles I'd never seen; and another chair to entertain guests. This chair had cigarette burns on the seat around an ashtray towering in butts. A glass of water, a pack of cigarettes, a lighter and a cordless phone shared the space and lay within reach from the bed.

Our patient was breathing, conscious, and sitting on the edge of his bed without obvious pressing issues. He also did not appear to currently possess a shotgun or rocket launcher. His elbows on his knees seemed to be what held his body up. Wiry and pale from too much inside living, he generally appeared to be falling apart. He didn't look up as he fingered a smoldering cigarette.

I brought up my first issue.

"Can you put the cigarette out? I'm allergic to the smoke."

Giving a medical reason gave less excuse to those who would keep smoking just to bother me.

He stabbed the cigarette into the tower of butts. Several fell off and became part of the circle around the ashtray.

I started again.

"So, what brings us here tonight?"

Without even raising his head, he muttered, "I want to go to the hospital."

I asked calmly in return, "Why do you want us to take you to the hospital?"

He sat up, anger flashing in his eyes.

"Are you officers refusing to take me to the hospital?"

I stiffened at his change in attitude.

"No. No one's refusing you transport. I'm asking why you want us to take you."

He grabbed the glass of water and slugged down a wash. There was more than water in the glass. There were floaties. Ew. He replaced the glass to the chair with more force than necessary then glared at us again.

"When is the ambulance getting here? You officers are refusing my request for service."

Okay. Confirmed. This guy resided in the weird zone. It was time to wake up, time to concentrate, try to make him focus and for me to regain control.

"Sir, we are the ambulance. We are paramedics. What can we do for you?"

"I want to go to the hospital. You police officers are refusing to take me. I called for an ambulance, when will it be here?"

Damn, this wasn't going to be an easy into-the-apartment, out-of-the apartment call. I dropped the medical bag to the floor. If I held it much longer I would have to either lean farther sideways to make up for the weight or tolerate displacing my collarbone.

It was still my turn to talk to this guy. James leaned against the open door waiting to see my next move, or he was sleeping, hard to tell.

I tried another approach and squatted down. This took out the aggressive, above view. I kept one arm on my front knee to protect my face. My weight centered on my back leg, allowing me to stand and spring backward at any moment. I used my quiet voice.

"Sir, we are the ambulance. We heard you were trying to kill yourself. What was that about?"

I skipped over the touchy-feely, squeamish words. This guy knew if he was trying to commit suicide. If not, the shocking words about killing himself would scare him and we could clear this up.

He said, while looking at the floor, "I had to say something to make you guys come get me."

A swirl of irritation passed through my stomach. I hated being used.

"Sir, what's your name?" Still in a polite tone, although I found it hard through gritted teeth.

"Robert. Robert Bellows," He mumbled.

Robert sat with his hands draped into his lap, head hanging down.

Suddenly, his head snapped back up.

"When is the ambulance going to get here? I want to go to the hospital!"

I yelled back.

"I still don't know why you want to go to the hospital!"

He was irritating me, sucking me into his game.

Robert continued.

"Maybe I will kill myself."

My stomach did another twist. I hated when people said that. I was legally bound to believe him and take him to the hospital. I tried calling his bluff.

"How ya going to do it?"

He sat, his elbows still on his knees. To the floor he said, "Razor blades. I'll cut myself."

Damn, the man had a plan. If there's a plan, they're more likely to go through with it.

"I'm not going with you two. I'm waiting on the ambulance."

He obviously thought we were cops. I was having trouble getting him off this idea. Also, I could forget the thought of leaving him. Willing to call 911 to say he wanted to commit suicide, he kept to his story and said it to me. It was time to figure out what made this guy tick, find his trigger points and develop an exit plan.

"So, when you called 911, what did you want the ambulance for?"

"Listen. You two get out."

He became more agitated, rocking back and forth on his bed. He rummaged around on his chair and picked up the pack of cigarettes.

This was going in the wrong direction.

"Hey, don't light a cigarette."

My voice was a little stronger now.

"Fuck you. If you guys aren't going to take me, I'll wait on the ambulance."

He played with the cigarette pack in his hands before tossing it back on the chair. He spoke to the floor.

"Somebody's gotta take me to the hospital. If they don't, I'll have to go to the ATM, take out money, and go buy groceries by myself."

I almost exploded. That's what this is about? This little pipsqueak called 911 because he wanted groceries? Now, I was furious, but he was still one step ahead of me. He had the phone in his hand.

"Hello? Hello, 911? Yes, I called for an ambulance. When is it going to get here?"

"Give me that."

I reached over and took the phone away from him to talk to my own dispatcher.

"Hello?"

The dispatcher, hearing another voice, asked me, "Is everything all right?"

"Hi, this is Eighty-eight. We're fine. Can you see about getting the cops here? This guy thinks we're the police. He needs a psych eval."

I tossed the phone to the bed.

If the cops showed up, we could hand him off to them. He still didn't need an ambulance and the cops could take him to Psych Emergency as well as we could. They even had the caged car.

I still needed some vital signs.

"I would like to take your pulse. Can I do that?"

I scooted a little closer and slowly took his wrist. He didn't pull away. After fifteen seconds I multiplied by four and called out my answer, "Ninety-six," and shifted back to where I started.

Behind me James scribbled information as it became available and filled in the standard sections of the patient care record for me.

Well, that went well. I survived and Robert didn't come unglued. Let's try another one.

"Now, can I take your blood pressure?"

I was just taking a palpated pressure. I was not sticking a stethoscope in my ears to have him blow out my eardrums.

I scooted back in with the cuff in my hand.

He jumped up.

"Where's the damn ambulance?"

I shot straight up and backed toward the door.

He was not coming at me so I stayed inside the room.

"Sit down!" I spoke sharply. "Don't jump up like that. It makes the medic nervous. If you make the medic nervous, he gets cranky!"

Robert sat back down on the bed and grabbed the phone again. He only needed to hit redial.

"Where's my ambulance?"

"Give me the damn phone."

I reached over, taking the phone from him.

The dispatcher asked, "What's going on?"

"Our man is a little impatient. Where are the cops?"

"They're on the way," she said in a tone far too relaxed for how I felt.

This time I pocketed the phone. Enough of this calling 911 crap.

Robert pulled a cigarette out of the pack. I couldn't seem to keep up with this guy. He was like trying to follow a toddler, lightning quick.

"I said no smoking."

I stepped over and grabbed the lighter off the chair. I didn't want him to have flaming objects.

Robert rummaged in the linen on the bed and uncovered a corded phone. Why did this guy have two phones in a closet of a room like this? He was beginning to piss me off as he finished dialing 911. They needed to make the number longer.

This time I didn't care what he had to say. I stepped over and pushed the button down to hang up the phone.

"Knock it off," I said.

I stepped back and he half swung in my direction. He missed. Robert was getting out of hand. I had to slow him down enough to halt his frantic behavior.

First, I needed to stop his ability to call 911. I took the cordless phone out of my pocket and pressed the 'Talk' button. I heard the dial tone. If I kept Robert away from his end long enough, it would go dead and that little problem would be solved.

"Hey, Robert. When did you last visit the hospital?"

He wanted to go to the hospital so bad, maybe he wanted to talk about it.

Robert fiddled with the cigarette pack. I didn't mind. I held the lighter. He tossed them back on the chair and turned back to the phone.

Damn, not enough time.

I stepped back in and put my finger on the button to keep it disconnected. I searched for the handset in the jumble of sheets and blankets. That's when Robert Bellows went crashing past my left shoulder and on to the bed with James on top of him. They struggled a little and James won by putting his knee in the center of Robert's back. He took the glass ashtray out of Robert's hand.

James casually informed me, "He started to take a swing at you."

"Thanks for noticing."

"Not a problem."

I turned my head and saw the supervisor standing in the doorway, arms crossed, as he evaluated the scene.

"Gentlemen."

James was a little busy making sure our man couldn't get up so I answered.

"Hi Stan. Good of you to drop by. Who called you?"

"Well, when a patient is calling 911 several times while one of my crews is in the room, that is something I like to check out."

Stan gave a little smile as he surveyed our positions. James's knee rested between Robert's shoulder blades while he held an arm so it didn't flail too much. I lay halfway underneath our patient and on the other arm.

"It seems you two might need a stair chair to carry this guy out. I'll go retrieve one."

"Thanks, Stan."

My voice was chipper. I liked Stan. He was a good supervisor. He didn't get all anxious and hot-headed until necessary.

We had this under control. James had his knee in Robert's back. It wasn't hurting him. It just kept him from getting up. Me? I was having fun. This woke me up a little.

I crawled out from under Robert. We kept restraints in the bag. I stepped over, pulled them from the outside pocket and spent the next few minutes tying one to each of his extremities. Robert, in the meantime, expressed his love for us. Well, maybe not in so many words.

Soon we had our man trussed up for delivery. The stair chair had a feature and could be flipped open and used like a hand cart if the patient wouldn't cooperate by sitting. We tied Robert securely, covered him with a blanket, and belted him in. I lifted the handles and rolled Robert down the hall. I felt like I was making a delivery and should be wearing a brown shirt and shorts.

Next was the elevator. There was only room for Robert and me. I stood him straight up, still tied to the flattened-out chair and facing the back wall. He still used choice words and now talked about my mother. He just didn't know the woman.

James smiled at me as he let the gate slide shut.

"You got this?"

Like you're really giving me a choice?

"Yeah, my best bud and I need some quiet time. I'll meet you downstairs."

I turned and stabbed the button for the lobby. Robert did a nasal spray as we descended.

On the way down I had time to think and realized something about this hotel and its residents. As we rolled merrily down the hall, no one stuck their head out as we passed. I know we made enough noise to wake the dead. Nobody cared, too drugged out, seen it all before? I didn't know. Who cared? It was three-thirty in the morning.

CHAPTER 21

The Bleed

"Eighty-eight, copy Code 3."

Dispatch broke the quiet hum of the engine as James drove us back downtown.

Damn it.

I was tired. Deep, deep inside tired; the night shift was chewing me up. Tonight my legs were missing important chunks. Last night it was my chest.

I grabbed the mike clipped to my shoulder and pressed the key.

"Eighty-eight, 23rd and Potrero."

"Eighty-eight, Code 3 to 2872 21st Street for the bleed. Police found somebody on the fourth floor. On 4-2-6."

"Eighty-eight copies. 2872 21st, on 4-2-6. En route." I unkeyed the mike. This time I said it out loud.

"Damn."

Four in the morning and dispatched on our twelfth call. James flipped on the lights, pulled a couple of lefts and rights to 21st Street and stopped behind the police cruiser.

I have to get more sleep. Tomorrow, definitely tomorrow.

I finished pulling on my gloves, got out and grabbed the blue bag. *The heart monitor?* No, but I did take the oxygen bag. One could bleed enough that extra oxygen could be useful. Good. The two bags only added about fifty pounds to my walk up some shitty set of stairs. James carried the clipboard and the stair chair.

The stair chair was a wonderful device that folded up nicely to be carried by a strap over one's back. The operator released the straps and performed Houdini-like flips to produce one certified chair with handles and seat belts.

In San Francisco there are hills. Kansas locals would take mountaineering classes on those hills. In SF we bought groceries on them. Due to the hills and the maximum stuffage factor of people per square inch in the city, I was forever doomed to step out of the ambulance, go upstairs, and carry my patients to the street.

The fire guys, who came blazing down the street while I made my bag selections, parked and crawled out of their seats with their own medical bag. We all filed into the hotel and began clomping up the stairs, rising through the latest version of rundown squalor.

I hated these hotels. Walk-ups, they called them. I would guess because the frill of an elevator was never considered, thus dooming the four floors of this filthy place to people who can't afford elevators.

As we rose out of the dark foyer, probably not improved with lighting, the six of us sounded like rhythmic elephants pounding up the bare and worn wood of the steps. The two bags over my shoulders didn't fit in the stairwell, forcing me to climb sideways and switch my view at each landing.

First, by chance, I chose to face the wall. Several layers of brown paint, slathered on within the last decade, added gloom above the formerly white molding.

I arrived at the landing. Switched views. Exercised the right leg.

Now I had the view of a handrail. More layers of white paint. Most of that, however, rubbed smooth and dark. Not to the wood, who knew at what level of Kelly-Moore that began, but embedded with black. The shiny slickness of thousands of filthy hands sliding down the stair rail, struggling to keep the rest of some drugged-out or drunken body upright, infected every inch.

The six of us, those with free hands, used that stair rail to haul ourselves to the next landing.

How many of these fucking stairs do we climb a night? How many in a week?

The anger rose within my belly and my head swam in confusion and exhaustion. I began an all-too-frequent internal monologue.

It is four in the morning. I am supposed to be sleeping.

Next landing, switched views. Back to the wall.

No, I am carrying fifty pounds of shit up a narrow staircase for some cretin who doesn't know how to stuff a rag on a cut.

Lifted the boot. Lifted the body. I lost my balance but pushed myself back up by shoving the bag into the wall.

This cop better have something impressive to say.

Third floor. One more to go. Switched views. Oh, goody. The railing again with years of skank embedded inside.

Now, wait a minute, the pacifist side spoke. *This cop's only doing his job. Do not judge until you have all the facts.*

And then bite his head off, countered my sleep-deprived attack side.

Clomping steel-toed boots at four in the morning kept the cadence of my internal chat.

I hated these walk-ups.

Oh, and it was always the top floor. That was pretty much the law. In fact, every paramedic knows the Hundred Pound Rule: For every one hundred pounds the patient weighs, they live another floor above the street.

This sucks.

I stepped onto the fourth floor and finally took a deep breath not interrupted by fifty pounds of bags pulling me back down the stairs.

Winded and sweating, I made my way to the center of the long hallway where an officer squatted next to an open door. Camp was set up at the hall's communal shower. We weren't in Europe and the idea of a communal anything in this part of town made my skin crawl.

Being the one in charge, I had to be awake. I stepped to the front of our little cadre, dropped the jump kit and oxygen bag near the cop and squatted down next to him. Everyone else stopped in a line and slept against the wall.

The officer knelt next to a fully-dressed woman sitting on the shower floor. I took a quick glance at her. She sat upright which told me her level of consciousness was good.

One guy, however, had died on the toilet completely unsupported. He achieved perfect equilibrium and died. I called my partner in on that one.

Tonight, though, this lady had color to her face, at least what could be seen in the dim light of the hallway.

Now it was time to listen to this officer's story and find out why he dragged us all here at this fine hour of the morning. I was actually a big blow-hard. In my mind I grumbled and cussed and threw vile curses at whoever created the reason to wake me up. Put me in front of the caller? Well . . .

I began with one of my standard openers.

"So, what's going on?"

His voice was quiet and soothing. "I don't know." His eyes never left the lady.

I was sold. This cop had been around a while and I was ready to listen.

He continued, his words soft.

"I was down the hall wrapping up some other business. On my way out I observed this lady in the shower stall."

He flicked a finger in her direction, as if to confirm which lady.

"I asked her what she was doing. She won't talk to me. I mean, she hasn't said a word since I've been here. She keeps staring off at the wall."

I shifted around. Yep, she stared at the wall. Every once in a while she blinked. Someone was in there. I reached over and softly took her wrist in my hand to do a quick guess at her pulse rate and felt its strength against my fingers. The rate was normal with a strong beat. Whatever was going on, she had a blood pressure. I still had time to listen to the rest of the officer's story. He continued relating his events.

"Well, since she's not talking to me, I started looking around to see if she'd been beat, or something. I looked for cuts, bruising, anything. Then I leaned in a little."

He leaned a little toward the shower, sort of recreating the moment, probably not aware he did it.

"I checked where to put my hand so I wouldn't fall on her. That's when I noticed the blood. A little blood is on the floor there."

He pointed at the floor. She wore a ratty dress bunched up to her hips because of her bent knees. I couldn't see anything from where I knelt, but he was wrapping this up.

"I can't tell where it's coming from and she's not talking to me so I figured I'd call you guys."

My knees began to hurt with all the filth-avoidance squatting. I stood to start blood flowing to my legs again and my back added its two cents about being tired. The officer still squatted and watched Our Lady of the Shower.

"Thanks." I said to the cop. "Let me in where you are."

My partner chimed in from behind.

"Hey, Scott. Do you need these guys?" He meant the sleeping firefighters.

"Let me take a quick peek at how much blood we're talking about here. I'll know in a second."

I squatted down where the officer had been. My knees had almost recovered and they groaned, remembering they just left this position. I peered into the communal shower stall. The moldy curtain hung to the side and, flowing below the knobs on the wall, rust stains formed an arrested waterfall. The whitish, yellowing tile was spaced with a dark grout. It might have been grout.

Sitting on the floor, fully dressed, my patient stared at the wall.

I tried the quiet approach first.

"Hey there." No reaction. Not even a flicker in her eyes. "What's going on?" Nothing.

I leaned into the shower. Gently. I didn't need her coming unglued.

No reaction.

I peered down beyond her dress to the floor and, yes, there lay a small puddle of blood. I leaned back out for better footing and also to pull the flashlight off my belt.

"I'm going to take another peek. I'm going to move your dress a little."

I leaned back in and pushed the edge of her dress back. Balancing on my feet in a half squat, I used the other hand to shine the flashlight toward the floor. More blood puddled on the tile.

Whoa! Holy shit. I screamed inside my head.

Aagh. I swallowed that one.

The beam lit up the four-inch fetus lying on the tile. And the red cord snaked back to disappear between mom's legs.

I knew where it went but, *Whoa! Whah!*

My partner chimed in again.

"So, what did you find? Can I let these guys go?"

In the few seconds I saw the fetus my brain took several still shots from various angles, including different aspects of the background. These "photographs" morphed into an impressive little full-color short movie.

Despite that, medically anyway, this lady was fine. She had miscarried but the bleeding stopped. For me to be nervous she needed to approach dead. She was not even near that category.

While some medical aspects to this call still demanded attention, the priority was this woman's mental health and for that I didn't need a bunch of onlookers.

I turned back to the line of firefighters.

"Thanks guys. We can take it from here."

Without a word they shifted and tromped back down the stairs. At four in the morning no one expected any "see ya later" niceties. I looked back at my partner and the officer still standing behind me in the hallway.

To my partner, "She's had a miscarriage." I felt a little nervous about using that emotion-filled word in front of my patient. But this wasn't a secret with her. I continued my laundry list of needs.

"Leave the clipboard and the stair chair. I don't think we'll need the oxygen bag. I do need a basin."

James grabbed the oxygen, heading off down the stairs.

To the officer, "Thank you for finding her and being with her until we got here."

I shifted around and rummaged through the jump kit, extracting the blood pressure cuff and stethoscope. With those in hand, I stood to realign my back.

"She's going to be okay." And then I added. "Thanks for the way you treated her. She needed quiet support."

He gave a quick smile. A second later he asked, "Are you guys okay here? Or, do you need help carrying anything?"

I realized we could use an extra hand when the time came to carry everything downstairs.

"That's nice of you. We will need help."

He stepped back a little and moved to the side of the hallway.

"No problem. I can hang around."

Now with things settled, I started over with my patient.

With her bleeding stopped the rest of her medical issues would be taken care of by a doctor, in a hospital. My job was now two-fold. One, I had to take her to that hospital. More importantly was duty number two: She should begin the grieving and healing process. My actions could mold those first few minutes.

A miscarriage is a horrible event and, while I had never had one, I imagined it as a shocking experience.

So far we were doing okay for this woman. The officer who found her was a good guy and now leaned quietly against the wall. He didn't take her silence as an affront to his authority. Oh, that happens: Medics, firefighters, and cops. He had been compassionate and quiet. I was not working upstream from the beginning.

I had a few minutes until my partner got back and there were things to do. Back down to the squat. This time, however, I put a knee on the tile edge. It was possibly cleaner than the 'grab it and breed it' environment of the carpet. Back to my patient.

"Hi."

I liked to be chipper. Well, not too chipper. At four-ten in the morning I didn't have it in me.

"My name's Scott. I'm going to take care of you."

Nothing. Not a flicker. Oh well, she was in there. Talking to me was not a requirement. I got over that years ago.

I didn't care if certain types of patients — like drunks — were unconscious. They could even fake being unconscious. I didn't have to make small talk with someone I particularly wouldn't be inviting to any family dinners.

Here I had an entirely different case. This woman hid under a major sensory shutdown to avoid recognizing her miscarriage. That was okay, for the moment. Psychologists at the hospital could help her through. I needed her to stay calm. I didn't want to wrestle anyone at this hour of my shift and several flights of stairs in my future.

Starting with her pulse, I took her wrist and counted for fifteen seconds, multiplied by four, and wrote that answer, eighty-four, on the chart attached to the clipboard.

I tried some more interaction.

"I'm going to take your blood pressure."

I took her arm closest to me and wrapped the cuff around. I put the stethoscope in my ears, pumped up the cuff and slowly let out the air while listening for the "beats." One hundred and ten over sixty-six. I wrote that on the chart. Her breathing was normal, about sixteen per minute.

I lay the cuff and scope back in the bag, closed the lid and forced the whole thing to clip shut.

We carry too much stuff in these bags.

I clicked my pen closed and stuffed it back in my shirt pocket. I was about out of little things with which to stall.

I could have filled out more of the chart, but it was time to stop avoiding the little problem on the shower floor.

Fine. Let's do it.

I had to make the fetus more portable.

This was one of those situations they didn't specifically discuss in paramedic school. The chapter dealt with the happy moment of childbirth and when to remove the bundle of joy from the umbilical cord. Nobody discussed how, when, or if, I could separate a miscarried fetus.

My job held many layers. Some of those were medical; others were ethical and still others were legal. At four-fifteen in the morning I was tired from working too hard and about to do a ten-second internal debate on the aspects of life, the sanctity of death, and whether I would get in trouble.

Why can't I have a job where the biggest issue is the stapler is out of staples?

I turned to reach both hands under her knee then put the flashlight on the edge of the tile to shine about where I needed it to go.

No, in my job I decide things like, 'What is life?' and 'When does it end?'

I moved her dress to the side.

Whoa! Eww.

There it was again. A little red chunk. Sort of shaped like a person. I had seen pictures in the news, the anti-abortionists with their graphic placards. I knew what I saw. But, *Wow!* Here, in a dark hallway in a filthy Mission District hotel, right up close and personal. Yes, that was the head, over-sized for the body. The back curved down, sort of like a kidney bean, with arms and legs.

Oh, yuck. Stop. What do I do?

The umbilical cord snaked back to disappear between my patient's legs.

I could leave it attached.

A visual of trying to move this lady with her miscarried fetus still attached played through my head. Murphy's Law would come into play. Someone would stumble, trip. Something bad would happen. The fetus must be separated from the mother and this was not in the cop's job description to volunteer.

Wait a minute. Another chain of questions started in my head. *What if it is still alive?*

A little jolt of 'oops' shot through me.

A countering soothing thought sauntered through my mind.

No, it isn't alive. A fetus that small can't survive.

I looked again and this time I faced the little red ball more clinically.

Okay, how do I tell if it's alive?

I did a quick rummage through the childbirth section of my training, the closest thing applicable.

Well, besides its size and the length of time we had been here, I had no idea how long ago the mother delivered. We took at least five minutes to get the call, drive here, arrive on scene, load up our gear and hike up the stairs. Add all that time up and there was no chance of successfully resuscitating anything.

Next. *Oh yeah, the umbilical cord.*

On a birth, the mother's pulse can be detected right through the cord. After the delivery, when the pulsating stops, the child is surviving off its own systems. The cord is no longer necessary.

I reached in and held the cord in my fingers. Nothing.

All right. Next step. Time to cut.

With what?

I did a mental check of what was available. The obstetrical kit sat in the ambulance with a little scalpel in it. The only thing on me were my scissors, which would work.

This cord, however, was not the size for a full-term baby. This one was quite small and soft, about the size of spaghetti. A full term cord is fibrous and thick, about as big around as a finger.

Why get my scissors dirty?

They would go back in my holster with blood on them and I wore gloves. The goal was to separate the fetus.

Is there a 'proper' way to do this?

I answered my own question by squeezing my thumb to my forefinger.

The moment was done. The objective met. I had broken the literal and metaphysical cord of life. I also officially crossed the line and declared this child dead.

I didn't even know if this was a child. It didn't matter. I had a chunk of human tissue, dead child, or untenable fetus I needed to make portable and a lady who needed gentle care to move her past a horrible moment in her life. I heard boots clomping back up the stairs.

When James got to our little group in the hallway, he handed me the basin with a small stack of Chux inside. These are great multi-purpose pads: Plastic sheets on one side, absorbent stuff on the other. He also brought some to spread on the seat of the stair chair.

"Thanks, James. Good call on the Chux."

He answered back with a straight face.

"Hey, I don't clean up what I don't have to."

Point made.

James flipped open the stair chair and spread the Chux in a layer over the seat. I took the basin; arranged a few Chux in the bottom, and saved some for a drape. I got down once more and, without taking the time to develop too much thought, I grabbed the fetus and put it in the basin. I took off my gloves by turning them inside out on each other, formed a ball, dropped them in the basin, draped a Chux over everything and put it on the floor.

I bent back down. It was time to move Mom.

I still didn't know her name. A tear slid down her cheek. I used my softest, most comforting voice.

"Time to go."

Her eyes finally moved and saw me. The tears held until another escaped down her cheek.

I asked her as I took hold of her upper arm, "Are you ready?"

I lay a boot in front of her toes so she didn't slide as she stood. I kept the movement going right on to the chair. I wanted a steady motion from here on out. We did have an issue that she might deliver the placenta at any time. I didn't want to deal with the mess or the extra emotional impact to my patient.

James and I thought alike. We handed each other the seat belt ends and kept a constant activity around her. I also didn't want time for reflection. We still had four flights of carrying to do.

I asked the officer if he wouldn't mind grabbing the rest. That meant the jump kit, the clipboard and the basin. I made it clear by our actions we were tied up and didn't give him much chance to get squeamish about the basin.

Suck it up, big boy. Somebody's gotta carry it and I kept you around for this very reason. I'm not putting it in her lap.

I guess he figured this out also because I didn't hear any complaints.

At the ambulance, the night air felt cool because of our little exercise. We lifted the lady in and got her settled. She still hadn't said anything, but she looked around.

I turned to accept the basin and the jump kit from the officer standing in the street. I put the basin on the floor at the end of the gurney where it wouldn't slide around. The officer waited while I settled things where I liked them.

"I don't know how you guys do this job. I have never seen something like that before. You didn't even flinch."

CHAPTER 22

Car Accident

On February 28, 1998, everything changed for the
paramedics working the City and County of San Francisco.
For 101 years the ambulance division passed between
different departments, but the world of the paramedics and
their precursor, ambulance stewards, was always two
people, two partners, against all the streets threw at them.
That day in February, for the first time, we found ourselves
in a bigger sandbox, being asked to play with others. The
official merger into the fire department went into effect July
1st of the previous year, but on that day we moved our
ambulances into the firehouses with many changes and
much to learn for both firefighters and paramedics.

No longer did we stagger our ten- and twelve-hour
shifts throughout the day and night. Like the firefighters,
we worked twenty-four-hour shifts and they all began at
eight in the morning. At DPH we went out of service near
the end of the shift to give us enough time to return the
ambulance to the next crew. Only one or two ambulances
dropped out of rotation and the rest of the fleet picked up
the slack. But with the whole system going off-duty at the
same time, the hour from seven to eight a.m. became a
pariah for getting a call and extending the shift until
finished. An amazing bunch of strategies quickly emerged
as we cleared the hospital and hurried back to the firehouse
without Dispatch finding us.

We no longer sat on street corners whiling away the
downtime moments of our shift. Now we stayed in the
firehouses, involved with the daily cooking and cleaning,
participating in the educational drill of the day, and
interacting with anywhere from four to fifteen other people
instead of one other paramedic. For some, this was great
fun and filled the day with laughs and conversation. Others

preferred the quiet time between calls to read or reflect and spend the day with one familiar face. Some made the comparison to cats and dogs. Paramedics can be cats: quiet, solitary, introspective. Firefighters are dogs: Happiest when in a pack, gregarious and team-oriented.

The firehouse tones, the be-bop, now ran our daily lives and heavily impacted the firefighters we now worked with. When a call came in, the lights slammed on and a two-step tone sounded, followed by an announcement giving the address, the chief complaint, and which apparatus was due. With forty-two firehouses in the city and only twenty-five housing ambulances, quite often the ambulance responded with a fire engine from another firehouse. In less than a week, when the be-bop went off, only the medics put down their forks and stood from the table. During the day this wasn't so bad. At night, the lights and tones became very obtrusive, at times flipping me in my bed from the shock. The department also chose to use the be-bop to tone out the ambulance already up and gone from the house on a previous call. This did not sit well with the firefighters.

What made the dispatches worse was an increase in call volume. Dispatch changed over to a more "legal-friendly" policy. Paramedics no longer answered phones and assigned ambulances from street experience. Now the dispatches were sent out according to questions from a flip chart in a book.

Dispatch answered with "911, what is your emergency?" and asked a series of identical questions for every call. The questions came from a laminated book opening bottom to top with tabs on the right side reading off different medical situations. As the questions progressed, the dispatcher flipped to another scenario which might prompt more questions until the appropriate level of response was determined: Only an ambulance for the simple medical calls; a fire engine and an ambulance for the emergent medical calls; only a fire engine for the small fires; only a ladder truck for the elevator extrication; or a full box response of three fire engines, two ladder trucks, three chiefs, the Rescue Squad, an ambulance, and a paramedic supervisor for working fires.

The old system sent out calls at sixty percent Code 2, ambulance only, urgent, no lights or sirens. The new system sent calls out at eighty-five percent Code 3, emergent, lights and sirens, and a fire engine with their EMTs for assistance. Better? Hmmm. Code 3 for hemorrhoids? I ran the calls I got paid to run and tried to stay awake long enough after my shift to drive home.

One of the best improvements was eating. We no longer ate out of to-go boxes with plastic silverware and a steering wheel in the gut. Real knives and forks were used . . . when we could eat. Each call took about an hour from dispatch to returning to the firehouse. The department was adamant we integrate into the firehouse and eat meals in the station. The record for running calls in a twenty-four-hour shift was thirty, and many paramedics saw wisdom in the old grab-some-food-while-you-can mantra instead of driving back to eat a meal two hours cold and getting another call when backing into the firehouse.

It didn't help that the firefighters had no idea what we did when we left the house. Their experience on the medicals we ran with them was a few minutes of the call before we released them. They didn't know about the rest of the treatment we gave, going to the hospital, or doing paperwork to high legal standards. It also didn't help when the medic would come into the house after the tenth call before dinner and say, "I need a nap. I'll be upstairs; wake me when dinner's ready."

Rather than find a bunk in the dormitory, some medics slept in the back of the ambulance. They'd been catching naps on the gurney during their shift for the last twenty years, and continuing the practice made the trip to the driver's seat shorter when being woken up six times between midnight and eight in the morning.

Every few months the administration would throw out

another plan on how they were going to reduce the call volume and move us to the fire engines, but many of the DPH paramedics quit. They didn't want to be firefighters, didn't want to work twenty-four-hour shifts, and believed the career of being a paramedic was going to be diluted in the fire department.

Not I. I liked many aspects of the new job, decided there was going to be no dilution of medicine on my ambulance, and twenty-four-hour shifts molded better with my commute. I'm also stubborn, can't turn down a challenge, and I never quit believing in the rainbow the department kept floating. I also needed the paycheck and didn't want to go back to my old job. Five years later I'd been cross-trained as a firefighter and worked my first shift as a paramedic on a fire engine. Until then . . . .

I could tell as we pulled up this was not much of a car accident: Little bent metal or car fluids and few stunned, staggering people. Coincidentally, the event ended in the parking lot of an auto body shop. I began finding out the number of patients and the extent of their injuries. The key was not to get tied down to any one patient until I had a solid count. I was doing that when I approached the car with the couple inside and leaned in their window.

"Are you people okay? Do you want to go to the hospital?"

It became obvious neither one of them spoke English. Their primary language was Spanish and I spoke very little.

"Okay? Dolor? Hospital?" I said with all the seemingly appropriate hand gestures.

They smiled at me and shook their heads. They definitely were not hurt badly and I still had to finish my patient inventory. I gave a reassuring smile and backed away.

"Okay. Una momento."

I turned to see what else I had to do.

I continued checking the other vehicles and their occupants when the Hispanic couple drove away. Seconds later a police officer arrived. I met him at the back of his car.

"Hi. Everyone is okay. But that blue car," pointing at the sedan pulling away from the next stoplight, "they just drove away from the scene."

The officer jumped back into his car to retrieve them. I walked up the driveway and met the auto shop owner. He looked at the cars (and the potential business) strewn about.

He asked me, "Is everyone all right?"

"Yes. Everybody seems to be fine. But that car out front, they just drove off."

"Do you mean that Hispanic couple?"

"Yes. I checked on them, turned to do something else, and they drove off."

"Them? They weren't in the accident. They were here for an estimate."

Oops. I could picture the cop a few blocks away somewhere.

"Sir, step out of the vehicle."

CHAPTER 23

The Cultural Divide

The tones went off and James and I put down our forks. The engine crew hovered in mid-bite, wondering which way the chips would fall, while the truck continued with their salads. They weren't first due on medical calls. The odds were in their favor.

"Unit dispatch. Engine 17, Medic 17 respond Code 3 for the 'Not Alert' at 1129 Palou Avenue #207, cross of Ingalls and Hawes. Respond on A3."

Six of us rose from the table while the truck crew threw out a volley of love.

"Have fun. We might save some for you. Call us if you need something done right."

A few minutes later James and I followed the engine crew up the stairs. We carried about one hundred fifty pounds of gear among the six of us and we all poured into the tiny apartment, filling most of the available floor space.

Our patient, lying on the carpet, was Chinese, somewhere in his eighties, and dressed nicely in a button-down shirt and matching slacks. His face was pale and still, his eyes stared, unfocused, toward the ceiling, and he had that dead look. Definitely "not alert."

I got down on my knees next to him. The rest of the crew readied the oxygen bottle and located the BVM but held back while I pulled out the leads to the heart monitor. We were ready to go gangbusters on this guy only if he was sorta dead or kinda dead, not dead dead. No use breaking out all the boxes and bags. Some of it must be thrown away and replaced, used or not, if opened.

I had the patches on, stuck them to his chest and flipped the knob on the monitor. The green blip materialized on the black screen and strode across without a hitch.

"How long has he been down?" I said to the relatives all gathered about.

A young man spoke. "I don't know. We just came home."

Official. This man was dead. Time to tell the family, finish the paperwork, get out of here and back to dinner.

I turned to choose my family member. The guy who answered looked like he could handle the news. I stood to face him.

"I'm sorry, sir. He has died."

The room erupted in wails and screeching and the family rushed the body. I yanked the leads off his chest, grabbed the monitor, and stepped back.

I'm a firm believer in letting family members grieve in whatever manner they feel appropriate. I can't insist my European beliefs are the only correct way to suffer a recent loss. I am sure many other cultures think us white folk a little weird because we don't express ourselves when a loved one dies. How many times is a family member described as "taking it well" because they are not distraught? Working in Alabama, I witnessed many African-American families grieving their loved ones. They are much more vocal, by and large, than whites. They kiss and hug the recently departed. The common phrase shouted out while screaming their agony is, "Lawdy Jesus! Help me! Lawdy Jesus!"

Not the white folks. They stand around quietly, restrict access to the body, and try to refrain from "breaking down" in front of others. They are permitted to cry at the funeral. The rest better be done after everyone leaves.

Not in this family. They lay on the man, cried and screamed, rubbed his face, and begged him to come back to them. Then they moved to what seemed to be the "we're going to try and bring him back ourselves" phase. The matriarch began chest compressions, well performed. She breathed into his mouth, all the while filled with sobs and plaintive wails.

I thought she hadn't understood my part in this. I went to her, put my hand on her shoulder and spoke above the cries.

"Ma'am. He's dead. It won't help. He's dead, ma'am."

Another family member stopped me.

"Let her be. She needs to do this."

Okie dokie. I took a seat in the armchair nearby with my clipboard. I had paperwork to do while the rest of the crew finished packing up the gear.

I had done about a third of the patient care report when I remembered I had to notify the medical examiner. The sooner I made the call, the sooner they got here.

I picked up the house phone and dialed.

"Medical Examiner's office."

"Hi, this is City Ambulance, Medic 17, Paramedic 877. We've got one for you."

"Address."

"1129 Palou Avenue, apartment #207."

"Phone number?"

"415-555-1212."

"What's the decedent's name?"

"Last of Lau, L-A-U. First of Chien. C-H-I-E-N."

"Time of death."

"2017 hours."

"Date of birth."

I stopped. I didn't know that. I forgot to ask the family before getting on the phone.

"I don't have that at the moment."

"Who's the decedent's doctor?"

Damn. Another piece of missed information.

"I don't have that either and the family's a little busy."

"What do you mean?"

"Well, they're doing CPR on the patient."

"What!"

"Yeah. I told them he died and they started chest compressions."

"We'll be there in thirty minutes."

Click.

Hmm, I might be in trouble. They overlooked the specifics on this topic in paramedic school, like so many other topics. They said I must prevent anyone from disturbing a crime scene. I didn't see that applying here. Technically, I couldn't make that determination, but I'd done this enough to see the medical examiner guys come by on a natural death and release the body straight to the family. I settled back in the armchair to finish my paperwork.

The wife still pressed hard and fast on her dead husband and moved, every now and again, to give him two big breaths, raising his chest to an impressive height.

Well done.

Soon, she stood, walked to the kitchen and put on a pot to boil, then resumed her duty of compressions. She sobbed and wailed the entire time. When the pot steamed, the woman poured a cup of tea, returned to her husband, and cradled his head to pour the tea into his mouth.

A new set of clothes was brought out and the family assisted in re-dressing the man. Finally the whole group gathered near the man's feet in a semi-circle. A camera preserved the moment with dead Mr. Lau as the focal point.

I finished my paperwork and the medical examiner's crew showed up. I didn't get any grief over permitting the family's actions. I didn't stick around enough to invite any.

A few minutes later James and I were back at the firehouse. The engine crew had caught up to the truck and gone from the salad to the main course. I sat down to resume my salad but I had to ask and directed my question to Wendy, the Chinese woman on the fire engine.

"What was that?"

Not one to let a jab pass, she put on her incredulous face.

"What! Just because I'm Chinese you think I'm supposed to know what the hell that was?"

"I was hoping."

"You're in luck, then. I do. That was the most beautiful thing I've seen in a long time."

"Huh?"

"The family . . . It was beautiful."

"I don't get it."

"You stupid white boy. The point is to show how much you love the person who died. The more you profess your emotions, the more you are telling those around you and the loved one how much you will miss them. That's why she screamed and cried."

"The CPR?"

"She wasn't going to let him go without a fight. She knew he was dead, but it was important to show how much she would do to keep him."

"Nice. And the tea?"

"You can't send off your husband to the other side without a meal and he should be dressed in his best clothes."

"Okay. The photo op."

"The moment was a very special occasion and the last time the man would be with his family. What! You don't take family photos?"

"Wow. Now it makes sense. That was pretty amazing. Thanks for explaining."

"Yeah, next time don't screw it up by getting in the way."

I could count on Wendy to never let me off the hook.

The tones went off.

"Unit dispatch. Medic 17, Engine 44, RC 4 respond Code 3 to 1629 Sunnydale cross of Hahn and Argonaut for the resuscitation. Respond on A3."

The engine started eating again. The truck never missed a bite.

CHAPTER 24

Tact

James turned onto Sunnydale at the same time as Engine 44 and we both stopped in front of the address. We were here for a resuscitation, a resus. I jumped out, quickly opened the side door and grabbed the blue bag and the monitor. James gathered the suction and the oxygen and we rushed across the neglected patchwork of dying grass. We followed the crew of 44 with their medical bag, oxygen, and heart monitor into the apartment. Six of us and our equipment stuffed ourselves into a small living room overflowing with a couch, a chair, a big screen TV and four family members, one of whom screamed, cried, and wrung her hands.

Bob, the engine driver, and Peter, the firefighter, yanked our patient by a wrist and a hunk of t-shirt from the couch to the floor, her head lolling as she fell. Once on the carpet, they ripped her shirt from collar to waist. Peter pulled his scissors from his waistband and cut her black bra at the middle. The material sprang away and her breasts slumped to the side.

My place was at the patient's head and I wormed my way through the bodies to slide into position. Once there, I dropped the ECG monitor to the right and my blue bag to the left, keeping my tools within reach. Bob rummaged in his bag and retrieved the BVM. He swiftly unraveled the oxygen tubing and tossed the end to another crew member who hooked it to the bottle. He placed the mask over our lady's face and pressed 100% oxygen into her lungs. James wriggled between the couch and the patient's side to start an I.V. The firefighter started chest compressions.

The engine boss did his role of shepherding the family into the kitchen, especially the woman sobbing and wringing her hands. I supported people grieving for their newly departed loved one; it was healthy. However, I didn't want them grieving all over my patient while I tried to keep her from departing. One family member seemed calm enough to watch while we worked. He stood between the kitchen and the living room.

I yanked the rolled cord from its pouch on the side of the monitor, peeled the white sticker off its plastic holder and stuck it to the woman's chest at her right shoulder. I followed with the black at the left shoulder. The red one belonged on her left side, below her breast. It was a long stretch from my position above her head while balancing on my knees. Her whole upper body rocked slightly from Peter compressing her chest toward her spine. I reached over, lifted her breast and slapped the sticker on the skin, trying not to get in the way of the compressions, or Bob breathing for her, and also making sure not to fall on the lady.

A flip of the dial and the green light traced, once again, across the screen, assisting me to make the same confirmation I had done only an hour before. This time, however, the dot at the front of the line jumped up and down until heading off the right side. The dot came back on the left and again bounced its way across. My own pulse jumped a little. Did we have something to work with? I had one thing to rule out: The action of doing chest compressions created electrical impulses.

"Hold CPR," I said firmly.

Peter stopped compressing. He stretched his shoulders as he sat back. We all stared at the heart monitor and the little green dot became the most important thing in the room. It traced across the screen and settled toward the middle. It came back on the left side as a straight line. Asystole. I was still ready to try and save her, but I had to be convinced she was alive less than ten minutes ago.

"Continue CPR."

The firefighters went back to work doing compressions and breathing for her.

I yelled out over my right shoulder toward the kitchen.

"When was the last time she was seen?"

A chorus of "Huh?" and "What?" rose over the sobbing and crying. I tried another version, this time without the sugar coating.

"When was the last time someone saw her alive?"

The man at the kitchen door answered.

"We all left this morning. We got back this afternoon and found her on the couch."

The official term was "unconfirmed down time." This translated into no chance of recovery and dead.

I looked at her face for the first time. Her mouth, still half open, missed a few teeth, and her tongue fell back and to the right. Her eyes, colored a rich brown, stared straight up and the pupils, usually finishing off the window to her mind, were now only two black holes. Looking closer, I saw the whites of her eyes had developed a pasty film without the blinking keeping them moist. I had only been here a few minutes but her face had already lost the emotion that radiates from the skin of the living.

Every EMS person in the room knew what happened and began quietly gathering equipment rather than making eye contact with the family. I often wondered when the relatives figured it out. Could they tell the difference between what we did during an attempt to save someone and when we stopped the attempt and started cleaning up? Or were they blinded by their hopes that mom, or grandma, could still be pulled back from the precipice of death? Maybe some knew what was happening; the others needed someone to tell them. I got up off the floor.

Grieving is a process and must be started to allow its progression. It was unfair and cruel to stretch this out. I searched the relatives for the head of the family or the one who needed to hear the decision the most. I easily decided against the woman in the kitchen. She cried and wailed in a small space while two others dodged her thrashing. I went for the man between the rooms.

The important word to say was their loved one had

died. I did not use phrases to dance around the facts. I did not say she passed on. I did not say she became deceased. I said she was dead. That word allowed no quibbling. It held unquestionable meaning.

I stood in front of the man. He was tall and the one who carried this family. I looked directly into his eyes. They were soft and wise, open and loving. I sensed the connection between us. In my throat I felt the weight of the words I was about to utter. He waited patiently. I spoke.

"I'm sorry. She has died."

His eyes said thank you.

The woman in the kitchen overheard and took her wailing to a new pitch. I turned and the supervisor stood behind me at the front door. He had arrived at some time during the call. I passed him to retrieve our things.

He said to me, "You guys gather your stuff and leave. I'll take care of the paperwork on this one."

"Thanks. Mighty nice of you."

Paramedics, most of whom never worked when this was reality, dreamed of running medical calls and not doing any paperwork. One of my partners worked then and I was his last partner before he retired. He told me of the days when he would grab the call slips off the table like picking up a fanned deck of cards. They would fill the ambulance with patients and take them to the closest hospital with no regard for their destination desires. The call slips were the only bit of information handed to the nurse at the emergency room.

Paramedics love doing the procedures; we love talking to people and solving their problems. We do not love spending twenty minutes to an hour writing a legal document describing the event and why we did what we did and why we didn't do what we didn't do. That document also must be hardy enough to withstand the scrutiny of a sharp-eyed lawyer three years later who holds all the information about the call, the patient's diagnosis, and the eventual outcome at their fingertips.

To have the supervisor offer to do this for us was huge and bumped him up a few notches in my respect book.

The firefighters had gathered their stuff and stepped toward the door. I paid my gratitude as they left.

"Thanks, guys."

James had also been busy gathering our bags. The family migrated out of the kitchen, the wailing and crying swelling to the others. I helped grab the rest as we made a fast exit.

I did a courtesy check with the supervisor.

"Are you sure you want the paperwork? I don't mind."

"No. It's okay. You guys clean up and get back in service."

"Thanks."

I brushed by and walked toward the ambulance, crossing the sparse grass, passing kids and adults. Paramedics, fire engines, and police cars were not an uncommon sight in this neighborhood.

One kid, wearing shorts, his legs dusted to the ankles from playing all day, asked while his eyes shone.

"What's going on?"

It was not my place to tell somebody else's business. If the family wanted the neighbors to know, they could tell them. It wasn't going to be me.

While walking away, I smiled.

"Someone's not feeling well."

We stood at the back of the ambulance reassembling our bags. A black Camaro screeched to a halt next to us and a young lady jumped out. She saw the ambulance and the knot of people gathered at her door.

"What's going on?"

Another woman yelled back from the apartment door.

"Where you been?"

The driver still stood in the car's open door, her question unanswered. She asked again, her voice rising in pitch, the fear mounting in her throat.

"I went to the store. What's happening?"

The response smashed across twenty yards of dying grass and neighbors.

"Your momma died."

CHAPTER 25

Christmas With The Eberharts

Once again we come to another Christmas Holiday Season. This year shows our family with fewer large changes, continuing toward many goals.

Scott is still employed by the San Francisco Fire Department. His cross-training over to a firefighter/paramedic is right on schedule and slated for May of last year. Yeah, the date's right. There's way more to this topic than room in this letter. He currently works Mondays and Thursdays. This might sound like gravy but, let me flesh out our common week: Scott works Mondays, Camille works Tuesdays and goes to school on Wednesday nights, Scott works Thursdays, and Camille works Fridays and the occasional weekend. We manage to spend a little time together, we tag-team our parenting of three children, and no one amongst our family and neighbors is aware of when we actually work.

Camille continues her ever-presence in the educational world. She is finishing up the semester toward her Legal Nurse Consultant's Certificate. All that's left are a few two- and three-day workshops. We're looking at the end of spring. Camille mentioned the other night, "Now I can finish my Bachelor's degree." Scott gave himself a headache hitting the tabletop. When Camille related how someone suggested she just go to law school, Scott had a seizure.

In the fun and frolic department, we continue our seasonal sojourn to the snow for skiing. The resorts have taken a new tack in redistributing our money by catering to the family even more. We put Kylene and Elise in daycare and for ten bucks more they'll slap popsicle sticks on Elise's feet and send her down an almost-slope. Kylene gets to play all day with new toys. It's worth the money.

This summer, in keeping with our promise to not go camping again for a few years, we went with the same other family who witnessed our last Tahoe experience and rented a house. This was a much better time with beds, a kitchen, and walls; things which make life with toddlers easier. We played Sorry, and relearned Parcheesi. Did you remember that game requires a lot of rules? Monopoly was another favorite. It was fun playing the old games and we all learned something about the loyalty of our friends and spouses and how to properly gang up on someone and appear apologetic while nailing their butt to the wall for rolling doubles.

Camille and Scott joined the local cousins and formed the "Quarterly Cousins" who plan an event once a quarter. We have had two meetings thus far. The first outing entailed whitewater rafting on the South Fork of the American River.

A recap of one exciting moment involved brother Tim's girlfriend, Beth. After navigating a rough patch of water, cousin Mary, our guide, informed us that because Beth's foot had still been in the boat, it hadn't been a priority yet to pull her back in. Beth had taken her cold water dunking rather well while also providing Tim with the opportunity to earn major boyfriend points by rescuing her, utilizing the tried-and-true technique of the front-breasted vest grab.

The second outing was a much tamer and sedate brunch cruise on San Francisco Bay, followed by running amok in San Francisco. The day was capped off by a play entitled "Shear Madness." The women got to shop while the men plodded along. The men retaliated with a perfectly sane trip on the streetcar so we could detrain and view the construction site for the new SF Giants ballpark. It was a glorious moment when Camille stood in close proximity to the piles of bricks, the chain link fence, and the massive machinery, and asked, "What are we doing here?"

Moving on to the children in our lives. Justine is eleven and has grown past the five-foot mark. She is running out of the inches authorized by her parents. If she keeps this up she'll be . . . gasp . . . taller than we are.

This year is the sixth grade experience and she's doing well as evidenced by the mostly As and smattering of Bs she brings home.

Justine is getting older also by the stories she relates about her day. It is less about school and increasingly about the more important issues of who is doing what to whom and how so and so is acting different when they are running around with them versus us.

But she proves to her parents quite often that she is smart by reading everything that doesn't move and continuing her piano and art lessons. She is in the school band, playing Camille's old clarinet, and is also in a modern dance class. The coup de grace for the year was when Justine entered three of her drawings in three different categories at the Sonoma County Fair. Justine won first prize for all three drawings. We were very proud and took note that she pocketed the $15 prize money rather quickly.

And then there are the small ones: Elise, who is almost four, and Kylene, at two and a half. Elise is thin and lanky. Kylene has no legs. We say that and look at Scott's legs, which ends the conversation. They both attend preschool, Elise for three days and Kylene for two. They love it. Kylene, thanks to school, is finally putting two words together, while Elise talks continuously.

They play fabulously when Kylene's not hitting Elise or Elise is not taking Kylene's toy or when Kylene's not innocently laying her finger on Elise's car seat and sending Elise into fits about the injustice of her space being violated. Those of us with siblings all have memories of bringing fantastic torture upon them. What is amazing is Kylene, only living for two and a half years, already utilizes a perfect poker face to communicate, "What? Who, me? I'm innocent."

But Elise also has her ways. She uses her seventeen months of additional experience to advantage, which brings us to this year's related story. Once again it takes place in the bathroom and once again while Daddy is home alone with the children. Maybe Daddy should catch a clue that the kids get away with more while Mommy's gone.

Having grown up with only brothers, Scott is learning every day about the creation, rearing, and processes of women and their precursor, girls. Every male knows about women and their predilection for going to the bathroom in swarms. It is a confusing trait men will never appreciate. Well, guys, it starts earlier than we thought. Almost from the day Elise had achieved her independence from diapers and was going "like a big girl," she would declare her need to go potty and search out Kylene to join her. It was innate, a genetic imprint.

One day this had happened, the process was complete, all paperwork done, and the children had resumed their play by staying in the bathroom. Daddy was aware (honestly) of where they were and generally what goes on and, hey, they were playing quietly. One could hear little snippets of conversation, but most of it wasn't anything more than the role-playing and turn-taking of their entertainment.

What usually happens when one can overhear a conversation, say, at a restaurant, is it is all a jumble and the hum of the atmosphere until something out of place or odd is said which comes out loud and clear.

Kylene and Elise were having a grand time with a discussion of some sort when Daddy hears, "Go ahead, Kylene. Taste it."

A mental inventory of the bathroom by Daddy found nothing edible which prompted his response, "Elise, what is Kylene tasting?"

Elise enlightened Daddy rather nonchalantly.

"The water in the toilet."

Another inventory of the possibilities produced two scenarios. The first was all natural but not a thought one wanted to carry further. The second required comfort knowing we do maintain a clean bathroom and the toilet is designed to present fresh water after every flush. A visual check assured scenario two was in action if Kylene had followed Elise's request.

Happy Holidays to you all and hopefully next year we'll make it out of the bathroom.

Love, The Eberharts

CHAPTER 26

The Delivery

A paramedic is trained to deliver babies. Doctors don't make house calls anymore and either some people don't understand the get-to-the-hospital timing or the birth is so quick everyone gets a shocker.

Luckily, the seven or so deliveries of my career so far were normal with no complications. I am trained and retrained to handle the emergency delivery of a child clinging to life from the first breath. I hoped, with passion, I didn't ever have the experience. My memories of baby birthing are happy. I wanted to keep them that way.

I did learn things along the way. My preceptor, the medic who taught me how to do the job, insisted I include the story of the patient complaining of abdominal discomfort. In my defense, she was petite with a small belly. However, she did complain of pain rhythmically timed every five minutes. My final clue was the baby coming out before we got to the hospital and soon after my preceptor let me in on the secret.

On another day I had some experience as a medic and I checked for crowning, the baby's head emerging from the vagina. I put mom's knees back together and proclaimed my assessment.

"Well, I didn't see anything."

My partner, Dave, crouched behind me like an umpire calling balls and strikes, confirmed his findings as well.

"Neither did I."

"Hey, shouldn't we check when she's contracting?"

Dave, playing the good partner, took my question, checking for flaws.

"Makes sense. That's when the pressure's on."

I spread Mom's knees with the next contraction.

"Whoa! Baby head!"

A few things they didn't spell out in medic school.

The other interesting aspect involved the cast of characters standing in the bedroom. Besides Mom, of course, my partner and I, we had Dad, frozen in a corner, amazed over the beginnings of life. Oh, and the Sheriff's Deputy.

After a successful delivery, dragging Dad over to cut the umbilical cord on his new daughter and packing everybody up to go to the hospital, I asked the Deputy what he was doing. He answered quite simply.

"I've been a cop for fifteen years. The call went out over the fire channel. Never seen a baby delivered before. Thought I'd stop by."

Well, come on in. Next time bring chips and dip.

Another favorite delivery story was the prepared dad-to-be who spread hospital chux (basically a two-foot square maxi pad: plastic on one side and super absorbent on the other) all over the floor.

"We're having a baby, but I'm saving the new carpet."

I liked them.

On this call, James and I rounded the corner on the "imminent delivery" to find a woman and her husband standing at the top of the stairs, suitcase at their side. I no longer tried to make sense.

I stepped out, grabbed the blue bag and headed up the stairs to retrieve a few basic facts, hear the story from the patient and also, to establish I was not a taxi driver. We would move to the ambulance at the proper time.

I conjured up a cheery smile and opening greeting.

"Good evening, ma'am. What brings us here?"

She smiled at me and her eyes showed no hint of pain. She gave herself support with her left arm at her back while her right hand held the weight of her belly protruding from her t-shirt. Nothing imminent.

The husband, a small, wiry guy, popped his head out from behind his obstetrically-enlarged wife.

"She's having contractions."

I tried to re-engage Mom.

"And how far apart are your contractions?"

Again, he popped out from behind.

"They're about five minutes apart."

Again, I attempted to direct the flow of the conversation.

"You know, Sir. I need her to answer these questions."

Once more the husband spoke.

"She's Deaf. She can't understand you."

Pregnant pause.

"Well then, why don't we all head down to the ambulance, shall we?"

I turned and walked down the stairs.

Mom settled on the gurney. I put away my bag and the husband climbed in, immediately moving to take his wife's hand. This wouldn't do. He couldn't be buckled in while still holding Mom's hand. Also, he sat in my seat.

I pointed to the back of the bench, inside the door.

"This will be your seat, sir. Please buckle up."

Dad peeled his way off and slid down the bench while I held the belt for him. They continued to sign to each other, his motions frantic. She seemed a lot more relaxed.

I buckled Mom in. Dad sat secured next to the back door. I took my spot in the middle. We were ready.

We only had about ten minutes before we arrived at the hospital and I needed this woman's name, address, phone number, and medical history. How many pregnancies and deliveries in the past? Allergies? Her due date? Any expected problems with the delivery? What were her vital signs? Finally, I had to check on the baby and the upcoming birth. I pulled out a fresh chart and started writing.

"So, this pregnancy is going all right?"

Dad answered quickly.

"Yes, it's been going well."

His eyes shifted back to his wife often.

I continued.

"Is your wife under prenatal care?"

I asked this question of every soon-to-be mother. I didn't know what 'prenatal care' specifically entailed. I could generally tell the mothers who took the classes, or whatever, and the nurses always wanted the answer. I aimed to please.

"Yes, we had an appointment three days ago."

He practically tripped over his words.

"She's not due till next week. Is she okay?"

This man needed to relax. He was about to experience a dramatic and amazing event. Freaking out would not help.

"Yes, she's fine."

I was calming a jittery, stressed-out dog.

"A textbook full-term pregnancy lasts forty weeks. But, anything beyond thirty-seven weeks is absolutely normal. Her due date is when?"

"Next week. June 13th," he said, still bug-eyed.

Dude, relax!

On impending deliveries I do other things so I'm not caught in a bind, so to speak. I asked Mom to remove her panties in case things started to happen fast. They acted as a net over the vagina, gumming up the whole works.

Mom did gurney gymnastics, stripping her undergarments as we rode, and I said, through her husband, "Tell me when the next contraction starts so I can time it."

I liked to impart a few bits of wisdom picked up over the years and the delivery of my own two children. I hoped it helped them, well, him, relax.

"Each contraction lasts about one minute. About thirty seconds of pain and pressure and they begin to go away. They may not be exactly thirty seconds but I'll count off ten second spots to help you through."

The husband translated while I spoke.

Mom kicked into a contraction. She moaned, rocking back and forth on the gurney. I glanced at my watch and waited.

"Ten."

I knew she couldn't hear me. It was enough being there for her.

Men throughout the ages know, at the delivery of a baby, they hover right around useless. In the last few years, however, a role has been etched out. According to my wife, Camille, an expert on all things female, a supportive assistant is extremely helpful in delivering a child. I would guess if that part is played by a loved one, all the better.

One may ask, why wasn't this woman's husband performing his modern role of birth assistant for his wife? Several issues obstructed that path.

First, I secured him on the bench closest to Mom's feet with a seat belt. The niceties of a cozy moment during the delivery of the child had been vetoed in a moving vehicle. If they wanted cozy, they should drive to the hospital sooner. Secondly, Dad-to-be was still not handling this well. He would not be an instructor at the "How to Be a Birth Coach" school for expectant fathers. Dad took it up a notch, wringing his hands and lamenting about his feelings.

Mom's first contraction was not a big one.

We were about twenty seconds in, Mom and I, with some moaning, holding the belly and light grimacing. Dad let out his own low moan and stated, "Ooh, I don't like this."

You ain't seen nothing yet.

So Mom tossed out the occasional contraction. Dad moaned and stressed in the corner. Mom said she had to go to the bathroom. Things were fine.

Well, not really. Mom didn't 'say' she had to go to the bathroom. Mom did some signing and Dad, from behind, dropped this little phrase on me.

"She says she needs to go to the bathroom."

"Huh?"

I understood, but wished he said something else.

"She says she has to go poop."

Back up. I knew this little trick. When a woman who is contracting says she has to go to the bathroom, she doesn't have to go to the bathroom, unless she does.

Women. They are out to stick us men at every turn.

Let me tell you about voiding in my ambulance. It doesn't happen. It doesn't happen because I say it doesn't happen. I have a short list of things which irk my stomach. You can bleed in my ambulance, in an appropriate manner. You can throw up in my ambulance. Give me warning to grab a bucket. You can cry, you can even scream. The ear muffs are up front.

Men peeing while lying down and anybody pooping? You can hold it. Oh, I have a urinal and a bedpan. I'm required to, the State says so. But I'm not pulling it out. I don't do that. Unless I have to clean up the mess.

Now, here was my dilemma. The bedpan lay under the bench, the bench I sat on. I would have to stand, lift the bench seat and retrieve the bedpan. This was not the problem. Dad was the problem. He sat, buckled, on the same bench seat. Remember him? Let's recap: Wringing of the hands, moaning and rocking, "Ooh, I don't like this."

I didn't like the thought of creating a loose cannon in my small space, with the ambulance moving and Mom throwing out hints she may be dropping child. Things were changing and it was time for me to limit my distractions. However, properly backstopping the arrival of a pile of dooky rose higher on my list.

Release the hounds.

I reached over and popped the seat belt from around Dad's waist.

"Stand, please. The bedpan is under here," indicating the bench.

Dad leapt up and bounced in the one square foot of space next to the back door. Mom threw out another contraction. Dad expressed.

"Ooh, I don't like this."

This wouldn't do. I told Dad, "Move past me and up to the front of the ambulance."

We did a little do-si-do and switched places. I lifted the bench seat, pulled out the bedpan and slipped it into place.

Well, I put it on the gurney, Mom raised her hips and I shoved until it appeared it would do the job. Let's remember, moving vehicle. The City still had street repair work on its to-do list.

Mom moaned a loud one and tossed another contraction my way. I saw hair. Not hers.

Well, damn. I did a quick survey of our situation. Most importantly, no, we had not arrived at the hospital. Two, yes, a head was emerging out of a vagina. Three, Dad still bounced, moaned, and lamented, albeit in a larger space.

Shit. Time to go to work.

I turned at the hips, ripped open a cabinet and pulled out the obstetrical kit, spilling it on to the bench. These kits don't hold a lot. Then again, babies deliver themselves.

I rummaged past the umbilical clamps, pushed aside the towels for containing the mess and found the bulb syringe. I considered this to be the most important thing in the kit; a little, blue turkey baster. Nothing fancy; simple to use.

A few seconds pass after the baby's head comes out until the shoulders follow. It also helps if the mom doesn't push at this point. The person in charge of birthing the little gem squeezes the bulb, expels the air and gently stuffs the syringe tip into the kid's mouth. The bulb is released and the gunk is sucked out. The procedure is repeated for both nostrils.

I was ready. It was time to take my position for delivering a baby. I also let my partner know things had changed. He was up front, cruising to the hospital and listening to the stereo.

"Hey, James."

The radio got turned down. "Yeah."

"Um, things have changed a little back here." I shifted over to the end of the gurney. "Mom's crowning."

"Do you want me to pull over?"

I glanced again out the front windshield. We were about eight blocks out. The baby's head went back inside Mom.

"No, not quite yet."

"Sure thing."

Dad bounced into my field of vision. Oh yeah, I forgot about him.

"Would you sit down?"

Mom moaned. Baby's head again pushed its way forward. I crawled on the end of the gurney, tossed the bedpan to the side and climbed between Mom's legs.

Dad, "Ooh, ooh, ooh." Wring the hands, wring the hands.

"Sit."

Bounce, bounce. I tried again, this time with more metal. "Sit, sit, SIT!"

Dad perched on the first inch of the bench.

Mom moaned. Time to go to work.

I crawled farther on the end of the gurney to lean on my elbows. I didn't want an explosive delivery. Tearing Mom's vagina has got to be painful.

Let's re-imagine the scenario with a math problem, shall we? Four people rode in an ambulance with ten feet of floor space, front to back. Dad sat on one inch of bench near Mom's head and, for the purposes of this calculation, didn't count. James still drove us toward the hospital and also didn't count. A chair took up three feet, then a gurney, about six feet long, leaving one foot at the end before the back door. If we put a mother, who is almost six feet tall, on that gurney and her upper body spanned about three feet, how much room was a five foot, eight-inch paramedic permitted between that pregnant woman's legs to deliver her child?

Too damn little, that's how much. I scrunched up with my nose right in the action.

"Hey, James. Pull over. I need a little help back here."

"Okay."

We swung to the side of the road.

The side door popped open and James came in. This acted like a trigger for Dad. He bounced. He never stopped

wringing his hands and moaning; that I could ignore. Now
he shot loose inside the ambulance like a ping pong ball
careening off the edges.

"Will you rope him in?"

James coaxed the man down to the bench and wrapped
the seat belt around his waist.

One less distraction.

James prepared to help by donning gloves.

"How are things? Do you want me to call for another
ambulance?"

Not an outlandish statement. Our patient census was
about to double. If either one of them had problems, more
hands would be nice. But, we were two paramedics and a
normal birth would be smooth.

"No, not yet. We're still okay down here."

Another contraction. This time the head started to come
out. The baby's face was down, like it should be. The head
came out at a good pace, limiting the chance of a vaginal
tear. I loved when a delivery went well. They were fun.
Well, for me.

It stopped. The baby stopped. Stopping was normal, but
they usually stopped at the neck, allowing me time to do
the suction thing.

This baby stopped early, at the eyes. That was
unfortunate. The nose lay below the eyes. Babies breathe
through their noses. This baby's nose remained within the
vaginal wall. I was now a little stressed.

How can it stop? What's with the stopping thing?

I ran through about sixteen situations at the same time.

Could I pull on it?

No, nothing to grab able to tolerate squeezing and I
didn't have any salad tongs. Besides, very slippery.

How about pushing the vagina back and off the nose?

I tried a little vaginal pushing. Nothing.

Could I go for coffee while leaving a note saying I'll
come back when things get better?

No. I didn't think so. People might see me leave.

The baby still hadn't moved. My brain sprinted through ten minutes in twenty or thirty seconds. Time to reassess the situation. We had progressed beyond a normal delivery.

"Hey, James. I think you're right. Let's call for a second ambulance."

I didn't know if James appreciated what I saw, but, later, he did tell everyone at the dinner table how I looked stuffed into about four feet of space and between some woman's legs. I knelt on the end of the gurney, leaning on my elbows, my nose not far behind my hands.

This was not my issue. I had relinquished style at this point to scrutinize something more pressing. To add to the fun, I heard James ask Dispatch for a second ambulance. Their response?

"Medic 17, we show you are already at the hospital."

What! My view of hair, baby head, and not-my-wife's private parts did not look like a hospital.

I yelled out from my little enclave, "If we were at the hospital, I wouldn't be asking for help, would I?"

The heavens opened up. My little problem moved. The baby continued its delivery to the neck and stopped.

"Don't push."

I was happy. I didn't care Mom couldn't understand what I said. Besides, I didn't think any mother was able to 'not push' at this point. I couldn't do it. Hell, I couldn't do this whole delivery thing. Thank God I'm a man.

I grabbed the bulb syringe I had, so far, kept out of the birthing gunk, squeezed the air out and sucked the mouth clean. Once more and on to the nose. Life was good.

Lower the baby a little. The upper shoulder popped free. Lift, and the lower shoulder slid clear. The rest of the baby whooshed out.

Dried the baby, didn't drop the baby. Wrapped the little tyke in a blanket. A little check for parts.

"It's a girl."

I ran through the initial checks to assess the health of the newborn, then handed the little girl over Mom's belly as far as the umbilical cord would allow.

I crawled out from between Mom's legs, still bent like a pretzel, and wiped the sweat from my face. I crept over to the bench and attempted to put my vertebrae into alignment. My back would be fine, eventually.

I turned to James when able to sit up straight, all smiles.

"We can get going to the hospital again. We won't need that second ambulance."

James shook his head, turned and exited the side door to go back up front.

Dad smiled and strained against the seat belt, too scared to stand.

We all arrived at the hospital, went upstairs to Labor and Delivery and presented ourselves to the nursing staff.

A nurse calmly led us to a room.

"Well, thank you for doing the hard part for us."

I smiled back at her, very tired.

"You're welcome."

I said my good-byes to Mom and headed to the nurse's desk. I had a report to write and then I had to get back out on the street.

CHAPTER 27

Epistaxis

AC/DC's "Highway to Hell" blasted through the speakers. With the windows open on a gorgeous spring evening, James and I cruised in the ambulance over to Eddy Street to investigate an episode of epistaxis, medical lingo for a nosebleed.

James slid to the curb, stopped, and I jumped out with a final air guitar riff performed on the sidewalk. In time with the beat now rumbling in my head, I opened the side door of the ambulance and hefted the blue bag.

I also grabbed the heart monitor. The dispatch information said this lady was eighty-one years old. At that age she got her ticker checked out for almost any reason. I swung the straps of both bags over my shoulders and bounced with the beat to the stairs, the lyrics still running with full accompaniment.

"We're on a Highway to Hell."

I took a position off to one side of the door, lay down one more riff, took my hand off the "frets," and knocked. I didn't really expect Grandma to blast a shotgun hole through the door, but healthy habits save lives, namely mine.

The door swung open. With no protruding gun barrel to suggest otherwise, I peeked my head around to find a woman with wild and uncombed gray hair holding the knob. A torn, ratty, blue bathrobe complemented her striped, stained nightdress. She smiled at me with a toothy grin, mostly; shuffled backward in her slippers, which would never again be regarded as white; and waved us inside her cluttered world.

I started with a cheery opener as I lugged our gear into the apartment.

"Good evening, ma'am. What's going on tonight?"

James followed with the clipboard. By the way, her nose was not bleeding.

She tottered off to leave us standing by the door and began her story.

"There's tissue around somewhere with some blood."

A quick scan from my vantage point revealed piles of newspapers, bills, and junk mail. No saturated tissues.

At the kitchen counter, our patient rummaged through a plastic bag. I dropped the blue bag to the floor, set the monitor down a little more gently as it costs $10,000, stepped nearby and peered over her shoulder. I spied a tissue, which possibly contained a tinge of red. Wearing gloves since getting out of the ambulance, I reached into the bag, around her scurrying hands and extracted the suspect item.

"Is this the one?"

Not seeing any others, I felt confident I held the evidence in hand.

"Yes, that's it." She hit me with that semi-toothy smile again. "I have another one around here."

"Don't worry. Let's go sit on the couch."

I headed over to the living room portion of her apartment, took the clipboard with the patient care record attached from James, and found a chair from which I didn't have to clear mountains of clutter. I set up in front of the couch while she settled in across from me.

"James, some vitals, if you would?"

I needed a blood pressure and a pulse. I would count the respirations. A recitation of the full story, then a quick exam would complete the checklist. James roused himself from his position at the door, popped open the bag to retrieve the stethoscope and cuff, and approached our patient.

"My name is Scott. What's yours?" My pen stopped over the space for her name. "Last, First" lay printed in gray relief at the top of the box.

"Betty."

I didn't write that down.

"Is that your last name?"

She smiled again.

"The kids around here call me Grandma Betty." Her arms danced in front of her, adding inflection as she spoke. "Been called that for a lot of years."

James rode a bucking bronco with the cuff wrapped around her arm. He needed help.

"Ma'am." She stopped flailing. "Can you hold still while my partner takes your pressure?"

James dove on the opportunity.

"Oh, I'm sorry. I don't mean to be trouble." She now used one arm to inject flavor. The other, the one James worked with, inflected from the shoulder. "It's just because my nose bled. It did earlier today and then again tonight." She finished with a smile.

"Betty. Is that your first name or your last name?"

I tried to finish one thing before I moved on to another.

"You can call me Miss Kay."

More light arm dancing. James put his knee under her elbow and anchored the obstinate arm in place.

"It's what my friends call me. I don't mind. Makes it kinda nice."

My pen had dipped toward the paper. Time to try another tack.

"Ma'am. Do you take any medications?"

I could at least get her name from the bottles.

"Well . . . ."

She slumped her shoulders, seeming to think with her whole body.

"Every now and again I take one of them Tylenols. Helps with the headaches."

"You don't take any other medicines? Anything prescribed by your doctor?"

"No. Never had to. Don't go to the doctor much. Don't like to."

Damn. That didn't work.

James stripped off the blood pressure cuff with a touch of victory in his motion and called out his findings.

"160 over 84."

He tucked the cuff and scope away and grabbed her wrist to count her pulse. I wrote the numbers on my chart, feeling a little victorious myself.

"Where's your ID? Do you have any of your medical cards? Medicare, MediCal, insurance cards?"

Miss Kay moved her hands to push herself off the couch. James was still attached and the desperation on his face was clear as he neared the end of his fifteen-second count.

"Hold on a second until he is done taking your pulse."

James finished, multiplied and called out the answer.

"84, strong and regular."

Yay, another piece of information.

I scribbled on the appropriate line.

"Now, where's your ID?"

Grandma Betty/Miss Kay shuffled off to find her cards. I spoke quietly to James so she couldn't hear.

"Well, this is going nowhere fast."

"You aren't going to need the rest of this stuff, right?"

Indicating the heart monitor and the blue bag.

"No. You can take all that back downstairs. I'll be here trying to figure out her name."

I turned back to confirm how our patient was getting along with her assignment. She rummaged again in the tissue bag.

"How're we doing with those cards, ma'am?"

"Couldn't find them. Wanted to find the other tissue to show you how much I been bleeding."

We were going to be here all night. The next technique was to do a little rummaging on my own. I started in the bathroom looking for medications. A quick scan of the cabinet found nothing. Off to the bedroom.

Working around the piles of clothes and knickknacks, I opened drawers and scanned the room. Not one pill bottle. Off to the kitchen.

I sifted through some cabinets and noted canned foods and boxes of cereal. I was also looking through her house to make a determination of how self-sufficient she was and whether still able to live on her own. If not, I'd call Social Services and get her evaluated for a nursing home.

I opened the refrigerator door. Nothing smelled rotten and she had milk which proved to be within the expiration date. The freezer showed she liked to go the frozen dinner route. There were dishes in the sink and the entire kitchen alone could use about a four-hour wipe-down. However, she had all the essentials.

It seemed she really wasn't on any medications, either. Impressive in itself for eighty-one. I also didn't find any ID cards. Next was the mail.

After finding it on the coffee table, I flipped past the junk mail inserts. Bingo. A utility bill.

"Betty Kay, 1211 Eddy Street, San Francisco, CA 94115."

The address matched our current location, thus solving the first name/last name dilemma. I retook my seat in front of the couch.

"Miss Kay. I'm all right with not seeing the other tissue. Can you come back over here and we'll examine your nose? I've also got a few more questions."

The newly rechristened Miss Kay turned away from the tissue bag and shuffled across the room. I wanted to keep her moving, occupied, and on task.

"Miss Kay. What's your birthday?"

I readied my pen in hopes of a quick response.

She arrived at the couch, turned, and aligned her backside in preparation for its reception into the black, plastic, fake leather cushions. My pen hovered, poised. She exhaled, supported herself with a hand on the armrest and bent at the knees, clicking through every degree of angle, all combined with a low groan during the entire motion until seated, and finishing with that flourish of a smile.

"I'm sorry. What were you saying, young man?"

My pen fell.

I could collect my pension before I got out of here.

"Your birthday. What's the date?"

"My birthday. Spent a lot of them here…,"

Her eyes sauntered through a long, slow gaze around the place. Half of a grin still inhabited her face.

"…in this apartment. Been here twenty-three years."

She focused on me again.

"Married for fifty-two. Fine man. Howard. That was his name. Howard."

I tuned out and lost myself in the stains on her nightdress playing the "Identify the Food Product" game by attempting to match the stain to the frozen dinners seen in her freezer.

"He was the better of us with the numbers. Kept track of all that. June 12, 1920. Heh, heh, I still remember."

Hearing a number, I snapped back to attention and prepared my pen.

"Is that your birthday? June 12, 1920?"

A thrill rolled through me. I had gotten an answer.

"Who me? No. That was Howard's, dear man."

My pen dropped to the clipboard and my head dropped to my chest. Miss Kay droned on.

"Was older than me. Always liked the older men. He was a striking one. Got an eye for that, too. Looked a bit like you. You're a cute one. Would have liked to take you for a spin a few years back."

My face burned and I knew I was blushing. I had just been complimented, rather brazenly, by a fuzzy-headed, gray-haired eighty-one year old lady with about four of her teeth missing. But I surveyed her eyes, caught that mischievous sparkle, and decided to take it for what it was—a compliment.

"Thank you." I smiled kindly. "Now, can I have your birth date?"

"Of course, young man. Just needed to ask."

Once more, the smile stopped her cold.

"And that date would be . . . ?"

"August 14, 1923."

Finally! I triumphantly wrote the numbers on the care record. I glanced down the line at any further information I was supposed to fill in. I then weighed against the odds of getting that information before the sun rose. Nope. It was time to do a physical exam, attempt to investigate the details of this horrid event, have her sign the form, and leave. James stepped back into the room and took up a spot against a nearby wall to watch the fun.

"Miss Kay. You say your nose bled earlier today."

I took out my flashlight while I lay down this initial question and waded into the waters.

"Yes. Yes, it was. Earlier today and tonight."

Okay. The hard part about doing a patient interview is listening and deciphering what was actually said.

"Were there two nosebleeds or did you have one lasting a long time?"

Two short ones, with the tinge of blood on one tissue, didn't worry me. A bleeding nose, particularly in the elderly, could be caused by high blood pressure. A serious risk of stroke. It was important to know which this was. Way too often I got embarrassed in the hospital when my story didn't match the one the patient now told the doctor with absolute clarity.

She smiled that toothy grin.

"Well, I had some bleeding today and then more tonight."

"Did the bleeding stop between the two times?"

No, that wouldn't do. I needed to be more precise and pick this knot apart slowly.

"When did your nose start bleeding? First time. Today."

"It started earlier today."

"What is 'earlier?' Is that before noon? When you woke up? Two o'clock? What time did it start?"

"Oh, I don't know."

"Give me a guess. Doesn't have to be right on, a guess will do."

"Oh, I'd guess about ten this morning."

Got one. Next step.

"So, your nose started bleeding at about ten this morning. Did it bleed until you called me tonight without stopping?"

"No. It stopped and then started again."

"Did it start again before you called me or was there another time when it started again?"

I was sitting in her living room at 9:30 at night. A nosebleed even close to lasting that long meant we were going to the hospital.

"No, it started again before I called. That's why I called you. I wanted you to come and take a look."

Whew. I think I had that one nailed down. She'd had two episodes: One at ten and one before the call around nine.

"So, when you had these two nose bleeds, about how long did they bleed? Were they easy to stop?"

"Oh, they bled. Kept using the tissues, but they stopped after while."

"The tissue in the bag, was that all the blood?"

"Well, I couldn't find the other one."

"Yes, I know, but were there only the two tissues?"

"Yes, just the two."

"And was the amount of blood on the second tissue about the same as the first one?"

Betty Kay stared at me with that smile.

The question didn't get through. I felt like a snail dragging each little inkling of story out of her.

"The blood from the first nose bleed, the blood you put on the first tissue, was that about the same amount of blood as the other tissue?"

"Yes. I don't like it when my nose bleeds."

"I can understand."

I brought my flashlight up and turned it on.

"Well, let's take a peek, shall we? Can you look up for me, please?"

She bent her head up and my light shone into her left nostril. Nothing special. I was no ear, nose and throat specialist, but I had seen enough noses to recognize no irritation to the skin, no blood, no clots, just normal nose stuff. I flipped to the other side. Pretty much the same view: Nose structures.

I dove back into my questioning. I could only find so many reprieves by examining a normal nose with a flashlight.

"Do you have nosebleeds a lot?"

"I got those two today. Didn't much like those."

Too vague a question. I had lost my touch with her style.

"Does your nose bleed every day?"

"No. Just them two today."

"Do you get them often?" That wouldn't work. "Do you get them a lot of times in a week?"

"No. None in a while."

"Can you remember the last one before this?"

"No. Can't say that I can."

I reviewed the extracted story to see if I had all the pieces. There were two short nosebleeds today with a minimal amount of blood loss. Her vital signs were normal. She didn't take any medicines to suggest a high blood pressure problem. She was a little loony but high-functioning enough as indicated by the fresh food in the refrigerator to be able to stay on her own. I was ready to wrap this up.

"Miss Kay. Do you have any thoughts what caused your nose to bleed?"

I wanted to piece together as complete a story as possible. Maybe she had some ideas.

"Well, this one finger. The nail is a little jagged . . . ."

She showed me the nail of her right hand first finger. It appeared jagged and needed a little trim.

I put two and two together.

"You mean . . . ."

I pictured the lovely Miss Kay with her finger digging deep for buried treasure. I sat back in my chair as the reason I was here hit me full force. Miss Kay called a 911 emergency ambulance because she had been picking her nose and it bled.

"Oh my" was the polite thought.

Okay. I had a few things to clear up and then James and I were out of here. I, technically, had to offer her a ride to the hospital. A paramedic cannot refuse a patient transport if they want to go. However, it was all in the delivery.

"Miss Kay. Do you want me to take you to the hospital for this?"

I threw in a little bite on the end to emphasize the last few words.

"Well, I wanted to be sure, you know?"

A paramedic is not allowed to give a final medical judgment. We are not doctors, but people can be pushed one way or the other.

"I'll tell you what I see. Well, I'll tell you what I don't see. There isn't any obvious blood or any blood clots. The skin inside your nose is not irritated or cut in a way which is evident. I know it was bleeding at one point. I saw the tissue. However, the amount of blood I saw is not a problem and doesn't worry me. If you want me to take you to the hospital to see a doctor, I will. But, honestly, I don't know what they would do for you other than look up your nose with a scope and tell you it's not bleeding."

There. I had offered her the ride and left it up to her whether she wanted to go. I could truthfully chart in my upcoming legal lingo that I had covered my butt.

"So, Miss Kay, do you want to go to the hospital?"

Miss Kay sat unmoving on the couch sporting her continuous little grin. I searched her face to deduce a hint of which way she leaned. Was I going to have to resort to Round Two of attempting to talk her out of this? Was I going to have to bring Betty Kay into a busy emergency room for a three minute examination with all the attendant expense?

She looked at me. Her eyes blinked a few times. I was drawn back to the stains on her nightgown. The brown one was the most interesting. It had little crusties allowing for layering while the rest . . . .

I stopped myself.

"Miss Kay."

"Yes, dear?"

"Did you want to go to the hospital to have a doctor look at your nose?"

Miss Kay closed her mouth and gave me a sort of sideways grin.

"No, dear. I'll be fine right here. Thank you for offering."

"You're welcome, ma'am."

Now it was time for my advisements to lessen the chance of her calling me again while still smoothing her over to put a happy spin on this.

"Miss Kay. Your nosebleed. It was caused by you sticking your finger up your nose. My mother always told me: If it hurts, don't do it. Same thing here. Don't do that. Your finger doesn't belong up there. Everything that fits up your nose shouldn't go there."

She smiled at me.

"Well, I didn't like it bleeding."

"I can appreciate that."

I gave her my best smoothing-over smile.

"If you don't stick your finger up your nose, it won't bleed again."

That sounded like it left a loophole. Better cover it up.

"Now, if your nose does start bleeding again . . . ."

Miss Kay jumped in.

237

"I should call you?"

"No."

I almost said it too quick.

"Don't call when it starts to bleed."

I was desperate and in grave danger of coming here every time she flushed.

"If your nose bleeds again, especially if it starts on its own, here's what I want you to do. I want you to take your fingers and pinch higher up, on the bridge of your nose."

I gave her nose a little pinch where I wanted it done, if necessary.

"Don't call me as soon as it starts bleeding. Give it time."

One final shot to put into focus why we were here.

"And keep your finger out of your nose."

I had observed her face during my little speech. She seemed to get it.

"Okay, Miss Kay. Sign here."

I flipped the form around and showed her where to sign indicating she agreed we had shown up and looked her over. It said yes, something had occurred, but I felt comfortable with her not accepting my offer of a ride to the hospital.

Miss Kay scratched out her name as I mentally pushed each of the eight letters out of the pen. She finished the last etch on the final "y." I whipped the form back around and, politely as possible, grabbed my pen back.

"Thank you, Miss Kay."

I stood and tucked the clipboard under my arm.

"We're going to leave now."

"Thank you, boys. Thank you for coming."

"You're welcome. You keep that finger out of your nose. And trim that fingernail."

"I will."

"Bye now, Miss Kay."

I started for the door James held open so as not to slow our exit.

"Bye. Good night."

She wished me well.

"Good night," I yelled back from halfway down the first flight of stairs.

In the ambulance I began charting my narrative.

"Arrived to find patient ambulatory in apartment, status: post epistaxis secondary to digital agitation . . . ."

CHAPTER 28

Low Acuity

0330 Hours

The lights slammed on, the tones blared out, and I did a flip inside my sleeping bag.

Damn. One night those tones were going to kill me.

The dispatcher's voice, awake and alert for her part of the shift, spilled from the loudspeaker above my head.

"Unit dispatch. Medic 10 respond, Code 2, to 2116 Turk, cross of Buchanan and Webster, for the medical evaluation. Respond on Control 2."

I strained out of bed and pulled on my turnout pants and boots while the other firefighters in the large dorm rolled over and went back to sleep. In a fog I lurched to the pole hole, making sure I was set before my twenty-foot drop to the floor. I landed successfully, stumbling away as Danielle, my EMT partner, dropped down behind me. We both staggered to the ambulance. Thank God she was driving.

We'd been in bed for an hour and a half after finishing our twelfth call since eight o'clock the previous morning. We had finished our dinner at midnight — on the third try. This was starting to hurt.

0336 Hours

We rolled up to the address to find the apartment complex gated off. This neighborhood had a crime issue and securing the whole area had slowed things down for the residents, but we now faced an access problem. A lady walking down the sidewalk called to us.

"Which one you looking for?"

I looked at my clipboard then yelled out the window over the engine noise.

"2116 Turk. We're supposed to go in through 2118?"

"Yeah. 2116's in the back. I'll let you in."

Danielle pulled the ambulance up to the gate. The lady saw this and yelled back.

"No, I gotta let you in here." She pointed to the walk-through.

I got out, grabbed the bag and followed behind. By chance, a returning car opened the bigger gate and Danielle drove the ambulance into the parking lot. She got out and the three of us headed over to the right apartment.

Escort Lady led us in through another locked door and knocked on the downstairs apartment. The door opened; she moved inside and started talking.

"Hey, Jarvis. The ambulance is here. What...?"

A yipping dog trampled the rest of her sentence.

This wasn't going to work. At three-forty in the morning I refused to enter into a verbal battle with a dog. Stepping into the apartment, over the dog's racket, I yelled, "Can you put the dog in another room?"

The man, Jarvis I guessed, herded the dog, a wiry, over-caffeinated collection of white fur, back toward the couch. The dog yipped and snarled, darting in and around, baring its snaggly teeth.

"No. He needs to go in another room."

"Oh, he's all right." The man continued to corral the dog. "He doesn't like people much."

Yeah. That was my point.

All I wanted was quiet. I wanted quiet because the barking crashed against my skull like shattering glass and I wanted quiet so we could move this along with little interruption.

Jarvis finally gathered Peaches, as it turned out, against the couch. The dog stopped barking but remained tense, quivering and ready to protect his master from marauding dust balls.

I was too tired to hold out until all my requests were completely filled. Peaches could stay. I stood, rooted to the middle of the apartment floor with the blue bag's strap caving in my left shoulder and mumbled my introductions.

"Hi. What's going on?" So much for originality.

"My arm. It hurts."

"Why does it hurt?"

"It's all swoll up."

He wore a jacket, so I couldn't see anything. He had been moving his arm pretty well earlier while chasing the dog.

"Take off your jacket, please," trying to be polite.

Jarvis shrugged off the coat without any problems. Sure enough. Below his left shoulder the swelling approached about a good-sized potato. An abscess. I stood in this man's apartment at three forty-five in the morning for an abscess. Abscesses do not start suddenly. They take days to develop.

I quickly developed a plan to, first, gather our information, then talk him into staying home, and finally leave before he changed his mind.

I dropped the bag off my shoulder and it thunked to the carpet. I flipped open the top and pulled out the stethoscope and blood pressure cuff. At the same time I fed my partner the info for the patient care report.

"What's your name, sir?"

"Jarvis. Jarvis Miller."

"And your birthday?"

"August 12, 1954."

"Is this your address?"

"Yes."

I stepped toward him and wrapped the cuff around his good arm. I stood over Peaches who bared his teeth. I shot venomous thoughts toward Peaches. We had reached a standstill, Peaches and I. The cuff hissed out air while I watched the dial and listened for the beats. Danielle took over the questions. She didn't want to be here any longer than I did.

"Sir. Do you take any medications?"

"No."

"Do you have any allergies to medicines?"

"No."

"Do you have any medical problems?"

"No."

Danielle's pen whipped through the boxes and columns, checking and writing the answers. I finished with the blood pressure and the pulse count.

"136 over 74. Pulse: 82 and regular. Skins: Normal, warm, and dry."

That was good enough. I could fill out the rest later. I put away the cuff and scope. Time to start the dance.

"So, Jarvis. How long has this been this way?"

"Oh. I don't know. 'Bout two days."

"Two days, huh?" My stomach acid roiled. "So, why'd you call now?"

I knew why he called. I had heard this very same story last week with the guy who ran out of his pain medications for his busted up hand. He called because it hurt so bad. Didn't know if he could make it.

"It hurts. It just got so bad. I couldn't take it."

"Uh huh. How'd you get it?" I knew that answer, too. He'd been skin-popping his drugs, shooting directly under the skin, and had a nasty case of cellulitis.

"I don't know. It just come up."

Whatever. I wanted to butter him up so I shifted into maximum politeness mode.

"So, Mr. Miller, are you wanting to go to General Hospital for this?"

This was my ace in the hole. The General ran a wound clinic. If he wanted to go there, even the Emergency Department would divert him upstairs when the clinic opened in about three hours. I was going to let him in on this and he would decide to go later in the day on his own time.

"No. I'm not going to the General. I hate that place."

Damn. Plan B.

"Well, sir, if we take you to the hospital, all they are going to do is give you some antibiotics, lance that thing and send you home. Do you think you can handle that?"

"No."

"Can't you take the bus?"

"No."

"What about some friends? Can't somebody drive you to the hospital?"

"No. I ain't got nobody with a car."

"Why can't you take the bus? This thing's been going on for two days. You'll make it a while longer. You want me to take you by ambulance to the hospital for this?"

"It hurts."

"Yeah. It looks like it hurts and should be seen by a doctor. But do you need to go by ambulance?"

"I'm feeling dizzy."

Damn. A nondescript medical complaint. Those were hard to step around. I leave, he tells somebody we were here and he felt dizzy. I'm in the shitter.

"Fine. What hospital are we going to?"

"Cal Pac."

That was the closest facility between where we stood and our empty beds. Good enough for me. I bent down to heft the bag back to my shoulder.

"Okay. Let's go." I turned to head out the door.

Jarvis stood and headed, most importantly, not toward the door.

"Sir, where you going? Let's go to the hospital."

"I need to put the dog away."

Oh, now you put the dog away.

"Fine. Let's keep moving."

I didn't mean to sound nasty, but I'd seen this before. I could sit down and knit a sweater before he got everything together and we actually headed out the door.

Danielle and I stepped outside in the cool, night air. A light fog helped insulate the quiet and the streetlamps set up glowing halos. Then I noticed: It was too quiet. We had lost Jarvis and we were locked out. *Damn.*

0351 Hours

I turned back to the door and applied a few soft kicks with my steel-toed boot until Jarvis opened up.

"Sir, we are leaving." I turned and crossed the grass to find where Danielle had parked.

I made it to the ambulance, popped open the back door and slid the bag toward the front. I stepped inside, then turned to make sure Jarvis was following. He was.

I pointed to the bench.

"There's your seat, sir."

I saved the gurney for the sick people. Jarvis sat down and I buckled him in. I settled in and started writing the chart during our three-minute ride to the hospital.

Seconds later Danielle called out from the front.

"Hey Scott, I think we're stuck."

Oh, yeah. The gate.

"Just pull forward. There should be a pressure plate."

We moved a bit, then stopped.

Danielle's voice again.

"Didn't work."

I turned to Mr. Miller.

"Sir, how do we open the gate?"

"You need a key."

"Do you have one?"

"No. I don't own a car."

Damn. This was getting complicated.

"All right," I played along. "Who has a key?"

"The manager."

The irritation rose in my stomach as I played Twenty Questions.

"And where does that person live?"

"She lives over there."

Jarvis pointed to the building behind us.

"And how would I find her?"

"Look for P.J. on the list."

"Hold on, Danny. I'm going to look for the manager."

0358 Hours

I hopped back out into the night.

Now technically, this was abandonment of my patient. I am a paramedic and I couldn't leave him alone with a lower level of care until I passed him off to a nurse. At four in the morning, with an abscess, I didn't care. I marched over to find the apartment manager.

I found the dialer and scrolled through the initials. Nothing. I even punched a few buttons. Anybody would do at this point.

Now I was getting pissed. I had an emergency vehicle stuck in a locked space. I was allotted a certain amount of time, about twenty minutes, before Dispatch started asking questions. To increase the fun factor Danielle spoke over the radio.

"Control, Medic 10. We are not yet en route to the hospital. We are stuck in the parking lot. The gate won't open."

I hated when my problems were broadcast over the entire city. I preferred to figure out these little things quietly. Dispatch didn't help. Their answer?

"Medic 10. Do you need a truck company?"

God no! That would be five more people, five more avenues to spread and embellish the story. Besides, the only thing they would do is break something to achieve the goal of an open gate. I didn't need that, either.

Danielle answered Dispatch, "No. Not at this time."

I wandered around the parking lot, banging on doors, hoping against hope I could find somebody official and awake.

I remembered Mr. Miller's dog. He had left it with Escort Lady. She was back in the apartment and, surely, not asleep. I went back over and knocked on the door. I used my hand this time.

0408 Hours

Escort Lady came out and brought Peaches on a leash with her. I dove right in.

"Ma'am. The ambulance is trapped in the lot. Do you have a key?"

"Well, yes, I do."

Hallelujah.

"Can I borrow it?"

I reached out for the wad of keys she in her hand.

"Well, I don't for that gate."

"And who does?"

"The manager."

Escort Lady pointed to the building I had left with the cryptic dialer.

I gritted my teeth and tried one more time.

"Can you take me there? Can you take me to the manager? I was already over there and I can't find it."

"Well, sure I can. Oh, and can you ask Jarvis what I need to feed Peaches?"

I was done.

"You know, ma'am. At four-ten in the morning, I am not going to ask Mr. Miller what Peaches needs to eat because Mr. Miller will be home before Peaches needs a meal."

I started off across the parking lot again, my gut now in full boil. My head swam from fatigue and I just wanted to go to bed. We still had four hours left in our shift and we could, potentially, get four more calls. Even the thought took my stomach up another notch.

I made it to the grass in front of the mythical manager's building, then turned around. Escort Lady had made it as far as the ambulance. She had her head inside, talking, I assume, about Peaches' nutritional needs.

I should have shut up. I should have kept it bottled for a little longer. I really should have.

"Lady! Get the fuck over here and show me where the manager lives! This is an emergency vehicle I can't get out of this parking lot. I need your help!"

Escort Lady stepped away from the ambulance and walked Peaches, his little nails skittering on the asphalt, over to me. She looked up and very lightly said,

"You need to calm down."

A voice came from behind and above me.

"What's going on down there?"

The manager.

I crawled back into the ambulance. Jarvis was still there.

We moved and were soon at the hospital.

My report to the nurse didn't take long while Jarvis stood behind me.

"Abscess. Left upper arm. Two days old."

The nurse looked at me and his jaw dropped. "He called 911 for this?"

"Yeah."

I tossed the completed chart on the desk and walked out.

0421 Hours.

"Control 2, Medic 10 is clear the hospital, available and returning to quarters."

"Copy. Medic 10 clear and available."

CHAPTER 29

In Search Of An Answer

Six of us stood in the dead guy's living room. He was pretty heavy, spilling off the couch in several directions.

With him being dead we didn't need to carry him downstairs in some crazy, heroic, and cobbled-together fashion, risking injury to all our backs and not saving his life anyway. The proper depth for chest compressions on him was huge and none of us could have done it.

I released the engine, finished the paperwork, and handed it to the medical examiner's collection crew when they arrived. Then I went outside and got back in the ambulance.

My partner put it in drive.

I picked up the paper again.

32-Across: Exhausted or made listless through overwork, stress, or intemperance, 2 words.

. . . Nine letters . . .

B-U-R-N-E-D O-U-T

CHAPTER 30

Christmas With The Eberharts

Well, here we are. Another year passed and we survived the Y2K meltdown. Spring sprang, summer bloomed, and Autumn is winding down. The Eberhart family is still here and, once again, not expanding but growing, thank God. We're all out of diapers with only some of us requiring an escort to the bathroom and that is only for company — no duties to perform. Score! Now, both Mommy and Daddy can say, "No, girlfriend, I don't do that." It's rather liberating. The joys of parenting involve small victories. Time for the annual rundown and then on to this year's story.

Scott plays the sax in bands around town and is still employed by the San Francisco Fire Department. In theory he edged closer to being a Firefighter/Paramedic by attending seven weeks of training during July and August, which did several things:

1) Exposed him to the world of firefighting and taught him to tie knots, lift ladders, drag hose, and properly make things soaking wet.

2) Allowed him seven weeks to think of things not even remotely medical. This is, quite possibly, the longest stretch of time this has happened in the last fifteen years.

3) Confirmed, without a doubt, that commuting on a daily basis to anywhere near, or in the direction of, San Francisco is a horrendous experience and should be done only to people one hates or while one is on severe mind-altering medication.

After graduating, Scott was given a new badge which says "Firefighter/Paramedic" and duly placed back on an ambulance doing the exact same job as before. As one might realize, this is only the Cliff Notes version. Feel free to call, block out a day of your time, and Scott will fill you in on the intimate twists and turns. Moving on . . . .

Camille is still proving she can carry the entire world on her shoulders. She currently works three, or possibly four jobs. It all depends on how one defines them and what parameters shall be placed. Besides being an excellent mother to three children, a superb wife to a special and wonderful guy, she is still the Paramedic Liaison Nurse for Santa Rosa Memorial Hospital. For those unfamiliar, she is the liaison between the hospital and those heathen paramedics. Her job is to teach them not all problems can be solved with tape and remind them they are not permitted to perform surgery in a living room.

She also picks up a couple of shifts a month at San Francisco General Hospital, you know, for the fun. And finally, she is finished with her Legal Nurse Consulting Certificate (don't get excited, she's not done with school). We were all thrilled, but a little nervous, when she got a call from a lawyer and did her first case review. Not surprisingly, she did spectacular work.

Hark, there is change on the horizon. Camille says she is working too much. She will quit the PLN job in January and go back to some ED shifts. This would mean she is only a mother, a wife, a Legal Nurse Consultant, a student, and a staff nurse at merely two hospitals. Ah, the life of a lounger. For the record, Scott stopped trying to keep up years ago and goes at his own pace.

On their anniversary this year, Camille and Scott went to Point Reyes National Seashore for kayaking. It was relaxing, paddling around Tomales Bay. The question was asked,

"Why doesn't anyone water ski here?"

We decided it isn't allowed because of the National Seashore status. Later, while relating the weekend to others, we heard mention that Tomales Bay is a breeding ground for the great white shark. Funny, that wasn't on the brochure.

Justine is twelve. For you math majors, next is thirteen. She just passed 5'5" and she weighs . . . well, she is getting to be a lady. The other day, Scott made the offer to find a large, vacant lot and let Justine take a turn with the car. She turned him down. That probably won't happen too often, or again.

Justine is in junior high school. She is assigned homework, time management is being learned in regards to that homework, and Justine continues to prove she is brilliant. This age is full of dichotomies. She is branching out to the books Camille and Scott read for pleasure while at the same time requesting a summary to make sure there is nothing inappropriate. She wants to view ever more adult material on TV but can be seen with the Disney Channel just as easily.

In January, Camille, Scott, and Justine went to Park City, Utah for skiing. It would have been better with snow but Justine experimented with snowboarding anyway. In July, Justine once again entered a drawing in the County Fair and, once again, came away with First Prize. She, once again, pocketed the prize money. Justine is also still involved in piano, art, and dance. She is quite the cosmopolitan.

Elise is almost five and Kylene is three and a half. They play well together and enjoy the game of pretend. Elise loves the game "Kitty." Kylene plays the role of the mother and Elise is the kitty. Sometimes they tire of this and Elise suggests playing "Teacher." Kylene plays the role of the teacher and Elise plays the role of the teacher's kitty. They also continue to make us laugh in other ways. Elise was in the bath and singing a song with the lyrics, "I need a man, man, man," while looking for a plastic person to ride in her toy boat.

They are both growing. They are measured against a door once a quarter and the progression is amazing. Utilizing a highly technical and intricate technique, by comparing the lines at the same age, it is determined Kylene is almost as tall as Elise. This is hard to ascertain using the real child. Elise never stops bouncing long enough to compare her to anything stationary. For this reason she is in gymnastics. Kylene is in the Gymnastics Apprenticeship Program, or GAP, which is free. She gets to observe Elise. Her turn will come.

They are both in preschool. Recognized as near genius they, of course, became eligible for college-level work. The choice was made for them to stay and do finger painting and construct paper art. We are glad the refrigerator is white as this is a neutral medium for the presentation of the many completed pieces. Throughout the day, the sun shining through the windows imbues the natural tones. This is juxtaposed in the evening with the harshness of artificial light to signify the angst of the artists.

For this year's story, it was going to be related how Camille conned Scott into buying a couch. It was going to be told how Camille wanted a couch and Scott wanted to save for one. It was going to be mentioned how Camille said Scott's family was coming for Tim's wedding and would be staying for Thanksgiving and there would be no place to put the planned guests to fulfill their derriere requirements. This got Scott to the furniture store.

The salesman had said it would be eight weeks until delivery, which, as mentioned, was the week of Thanksgiving. Scott acquiesced (gave in). The manufacturer informed the store and the purchasing party (us) that delivery would be in ten weeks. Note this is after Thanksgiving, thus making the original argument for couch purchase invalid. However, Camille had expertly utilized the "foot in the door" technique, which made it harder for Scott to renege without feeling like a total Scrooge. The couch was received after Thanksgiving, which, as highlighted, occurred two weeks after the household of guests left. Again, refer to purchase argument, paragraph above, sentence three. But that's not going to be this year's story because something else happened a few days ago which seemed a better fit.

This year's story happened when Camille and Scott attended San Francisco General's ED Christmas Party. The lovely couple got all gussied up and drove for an hour to San Francisco to Stern Grove, an idyllic setting amongst a small group of redwoods (cue music). Camille and Scott mingled and mixed while proving they were not the same person. Remember Camille and Scott both work at or take patients to the General but due to childcare, never on the same day. They then found a table and set about enjoying a scrumptious buffet which leaned a little heavy on the anchovies in the Caesar salad. The band began and a few tables were removed for dancing, including the one they had so recently been dining upon.

Here's the rub. Scott had used his keys to mark his spot and they were cleared away with the table. Scott noticed this and spent the next hour, while wearing a coat and tie, dumpster diving and looking through all the garbage bags. Did you know Americans throw away too much food? The keys were found, still in the kitchen. Camille looked at her watch and it was the time agreed upon to leave. A fun time was had by all.

Merry Christmas and Happy Chanukah.

CHAPTER 31

How Rude

Fileted by the rapid swipe of an attacker's blade, the man's neck gaped open. From under his left jaw, across the front, to below his right jaw, the muscles, tendons, and whatever else made up this guy's neck lay in full view while I placed my hands, one on each side by his ears, to support his head. It was kind of cool—if I had the time to poke around. I had an exam to finish, a treatment plan to devise, and I already sensed the pressure of an increasingly vocal circle of his friends who watched too much TV. Apparently I should look more frantic about this whole thing and I should be throwing our man, here, into the ambulance like a sack of flour to whisk him away.

"What are you doing? Stop messing around!"

There wasn't a lot of bleeding. More importantly, there also weren't any bubbles arising from the mess. That would mean his trachea got cut.

Pretty impressive and . . . damn lucky.

Dealing with a cut, there are several things to consider. First, control the bleeding. In this instance, not a lot. A few pieces of gauze should catch any drips. Second, what got sliced and what structure has been compromised? Surprisingly little but I was still too amazed over the view of this guy's neck to call it good and let go my hands. I would feel much better if I had help supporting the equivalent of a watermelon on top of a stick with the stick chopped.

I turned and spoke calmly to my partner.

"I need a c-collar and then just the gurney will be fine."

A cervical collar appeared, got wrapped around his neck and the hard plastic served the same purpose as my hands. Now I could relax, load this guy, and get out of here. On the way in, I'd start an IV. Other than that, he had a cut.

It was in an interesting place and needed to be treated gingerly, but I felt we were under control.

"Okay, sir. I'm going to hold on to your neck. I want you to stand straight up and sit on this gurney."

What he said next I did not expect.

"I ain't going to the hospital."

My stomach dropped. This guy put in a speed bump. On serious trauma calls, I hated speed bumps. I tried the light and humorous approach.

"Um, sir. You've got a large cut to your neck. If you saw it, you'd say, 'Damn! That guy needs to go to the hospital.'"

"I don't care. I ain't going."

"Sir, this isn't going to work. Your neck is sliced open. The cut is almost ear to ear."

"Nope. I'll be fine."

The circle of friends tightened around us.

"Take him outta here!"

If I didn't produce some visible action, quickly, I foresaw a beating. Mine. Only marginally less important was the fact that I was not going to leave this guy here. Legally, I knew, he could refuse treatment as long as he remained lucid. But, damn! His head was almost cut off.

"Sir, we are going to the hospital."

I called for the gurney to be brought in closer. I shifted around to the man's side. The man outweighed me by fifty pounds and stood six inches over me.

"I ain't going."

"Yes, you are." I pushed him back on the gurney.

I was amazed at what a uniform and a badge got me. In my street clothes I wouldn't last three minutes with the way I talked to and prodded this man.

Once in the ambulance, like almost every other time I played hard ball, the patient gave in and allowed me to do anything I wanted in the name of my job. We zipped to the hospital, arriving in about seven minutes, and I still had an IV to start. The equipment lay on a shelf across the patient from me.

I grabbed the bar at the ceiling for support, then leaned over to grab the tray for starting an IV.

The patient, still sitting bolt upright, with a stoic face, and his "man meter" revving on high, said loudly,

"Hey, get your nuts out of my face."

My response was simple.

"Dude, that is the least of your worries. I want this IV started before the hospital."

"Whatever. Just finish it."

I shook my head. Gee, what a charmer. Why did this guy get his neck sliced?

CHAPTER 33

Fire In The Building

"Box! 6-4-4-6!"

Forks crashed to the table and eleven dinner plates were abandoned.

The dispatcher continued, her voice clear and crisp, "Location: 954 Avery Street, cross of Tuscany and Willard."

I ran to my ambulance, taking off my outer shirt while dodging other firefighters who ripped off their station boots, dropped their pants, and stepped into their turnouts.

"Units due: Engine 42, Engine 17, Engine 9."

The rest of my uniform got thrown aside to pull on my fire gear.

"Truck 17, Truck 9, Battalion 10, Division 3."

Pockets filled with tools, my coat hung heavy as I shrugged it on, clipped the buckles, and affixed the Velcro.

"Rescue 2, RC 4, and Medic 17."

Bruce slid behind the wheel. On my side, shutting the door proved difficult with the added bulk of my turnout coat and pants.

"Respond on A-3 for Fire in the Building. Your tach channel is A-10. Reports are: People trapped."

All rigs bounded out the doors..

"Repeating. Box! 6-4-4-6! Units due..."

Bruce and I, as Medic 17, followed close behind Engine 17, speeding through the streets. Truck 17, weighted with tools and ladders, trailed behind.

"Hey, Scott, is there anything about the people trapped?"

I scrolled through the computer screen.

"No. Engine 42 should be there soon. They'll find 'em."

We drove into the hills on the other side of the freeway with tight streets and even tighter homes. One, maybe two inches, separated buildings. Fighting fire in San Francisco was tough. The fire must be met head on; it can't be surrounded. We must beat it down inside the house.

Engines 42 and 9 were already working as we arrived. Their hose lines snaked in the front door while another firefighter chopped at the garage door. The enlarging hole belched orange flame.

I dove into the throng of neighbors lining the sidewalk, scanning faces, looking for a clue, someone pointing me in any direction to an injured person.

A man waved me in with frantic gestures to reveal the woman slumped against him. I stepped in and raised her face to find it clean and relaxed. With no soot around her nose and mouth, I decided she hadn't been in the fire. She also didn't make sucking-in motions at her face, neck, or chest that would tell me she had trouble breathing. Something else was going on. I made a rapid assessment of her consciousness by speaking sharply, close to her face.

"Hey!"

She moaned weakly and didn't open her eyes.

Not good enough.

A chill ran through me. I didn't have any of my equipment, not even a gurney. Without my tools I felt stripped. Jumping out of the ambulance and diving into the crowd had been a dramatic, stupid, move. What now?

I stooped and she draped over my shoulder. I carried her along the sidewalk, weaving through a stream of arriving firefighters, back to the ambulance.

Once she lay on the gurney, under the bank of bright lights, it was time to reassess. I started from the beginning of my exam and mentally established a checklist of problems and findings.

My patient appeared to be in her forties, arousable by voice to a weak verbal response, with a clear airway, no trouble breathing, and notably without the dark soot coating her nose and mouth if she had been exposed to the smoke of the fire.

I pulled the leads from the heart monitor, slapped the stickers on her chest, and flipped the dial to start the screen. The clip of the pulse oximeter slipped over her finger, measuring oxygen levels in the body to give a saturation percentage, a "sat." Her heart rate appeared normal at eighty-four and her sat scanned out at ninety-six percent. Again, absolutely normal.

Something else was going on.

"Ma'am. What's your name?"

She answered, but slowly. "Gilda . . . Gilda Jones."

She wasn't awake enough for me. I grabbed a nasal cannula, put the prongs in her nose and spun the dial to four liters of oxygen per minute.

Let's see if that perks her up. If not, she could use it.

"What happened?" The urgency in my voice rose.

She curled on the gurney, her feet tucked under her, trying to make herself small. Trying to escape. Something had happened and she didn't want it to find her.

"Gilda, what happened? I need to know if you are hurt. Were you in the fire?"

"No. I couldn't get in."

I sat a little straighter. "Why did you try to get in?"

"Their faces. Right there at the gate. I couldn't open it. They were right there."

"Who was right there?" I leaned forward to catch her words the first time.

"The children. They were at the gate. I left to call 911. When I came back they were gone." She sobbed into her hands. Huge, racking sobs.

An image formed in my mind: Children screaming and crying pressed against the security gate on the front door which had become the bars of their prison.

At least twenty-six firefighters worked and searched inside or on the roof. The children would be found.

As for Mrs. Jones, she was fine. Medically anyway. She sat on the gurney staring at the back door of the ambulance while I grabbed a quick blood pressure to round out the normal findings of her vital signs and wrote the numbers on the chart.

"Do you want me to take you to the hospital?"

"No. I don't want to go."

"Okay. Can you sign this form? It says I offered you the ride. You can still sit here if you like."

She scribbled her name where I pointed.

"Thank you. No," she said.

As she left the gurney I placed my hand on her shoulder and asked, "Are you okay? Are you sure?"

"Yes. My husband is across the street. Probably wondering where I am. Thank you. I'll go."

"All right. If you need anything, I'll be here for a while. Come find me."

She climbed out into the glowing night as flames erupted from an upstairs window and the glass crashed to the street.

I slid out behind her and put on the rest of my firefighting gear. With my medical bag and heart monitor I headed toward the command post. My partner? He'd been gone since I got out of the ambulance.

The street in front of the house shone and glistened from the fire, the water, and the streetlights. Flames still jumped from the windows, but they were now chased by blasts of water into the night sky.

A firefighter stepped out the front door. He carried something. I couldn't see what through the bulk of his turnout coat, but I knew he searched for me.

I yelled and waved.

"Over here. Bring him over here."

I dropped my equipment as we met in the intersection. "Put him down."

The firefighter gently placed my second patient of the night, a small boy about one year old, on the pavement. The child, sprawled on the street, lay covered in soot and burns. My hands froze over his motionless body and I caught a cry in my throat as the smoke hit my nose. I tasted the acrid grit on my tongue.

No, keep moving. Move! I shoved the cry down.

I shook the boy for responsiveness. Nothing. I felt for a pulse at his neck. Nothing.

Two other paramedics came from behind, dropped a flat stretcher on the ground, moved the boy on to it, and, without a word or asking for a report of his condition, disappeared.

Not seconds later another child lay next to where the first just left. I grabbed my bag and scooted to my next patient.

Boy or girl? It didn't matter. This one was burnt like the last one.

Responsive? Shake. Nothing. Pulse? No. Another crew reached in and took the patient away. Another child fell to the pavement.

Damn. I swallowed the horror again. Grabbed my bag. Scooted forward. Started again. This one seemed about three years old. Burnt.

Responsive? No. Pulse? No.

Again, a crew dropped in, slid the child to a stretcher and took off.

A fourth child arrived. She was the biggest – twelve or so – and her legs hung beyond the grasp of the firefighter as he fell to his knees, released his hold and lay her on the asphalt. Her clothes were burnt and sooty.

God, I can't go on.

I grabbed my bag, shifted again.

Responsive? No. Pulse at the neck? No.

I paused, waiting for another crew to sweep my patient from me. Nobody came. I heard my own voice again, Move. Don't let go yet. It's not time.

Next step. I reached back and brought my heart monitor up from where I left it — three children ago.

I yanked on the wire ends, then stuck the patches on her chest, flipped the dial and waited for the green dot to show on the screen, showing me the electrical activity of this child's heart. The luminescent blip flowed unwavering from left to right. I double-checked the patches, then followed the cord back to the machine and checked to make sure it was hooked up right. I had to be sure. When I made this decision it had to be right and it had to be final.

The firefighter who brought her out still knelt on the street watching and waiting, hoping he had pulled her to safety soon enough. Our eyes met.

"She's dead."

He nodded his understanding.

No more children came out of the house. This last one was dead by my declaration. Still, I couldn't let go. I had work to do as the fire raged on.

I searched to find a place for my remaining patient. She was not going in my ambulance. Dead people didn't go in my ambulance. I noticed a bush next to the house and out of the way.

I said to the firefighter, "Let's put her over there. We can cover her up."

We carried her by legs and arms. We had to be careful. A crowd of at least one hundred, her neighbors, watched our every move. Another firefighter, thinking ahead, jogged back to us with a yellow blanket to spread over her.

I turned and gathered my equipment. A woman stepped up to me. In a raspy voice she said, "I can't breathe."

Oh shit. A fire scene, breathing problems, and raspy voices set off alarm bells. If a person breathed the super-heated gases of a fire, their airway swelled closed in minutes. A raspy voice was a late sign.

I look at her face. It was relaxed. No soot in her nose or around her mouth. I asked her firmly, "Were you in the fire?"

"No. I have asthma. It's acting up."

Relief passed over me. An asthma attack. "Let's get you back to the ambulance. I'll give you a breathing treatment."

We walked back toward the ambulance, passing two firefighters pushing a gurney carrying a child. It was one of the kids. I think the third one from the street.

I said to the firefighters, "What are you two doing?"

"We can't find an empty ambulance."

I glanced around and saw none available.

"Fine. Put him in mine."

The child had been taken from the street, laid on a gurney and just wheeled away from my care in the expectation there would be an ambulance waiting to receive him. That didn't happen and I now had two patients.

As the firefighters rolled the gurney to my ambulance a man stepped up to me.

"I'm a pediatrician. Can I help?"

Normally, I didn't take help from physicians on scene. By the time I explained the legalities involved in using their help, I might be done with my treatments. This time, however, I could use the extra hand.

"Sure. Hop in. Sit in the seat behind the kid's head."

I directed my asthma patient to the bench as the gurney carrying the child got locked in. The firefighters took off to find a new assignment. Damn. I could have used them. Until I got these two patients sorted out, the list of things to do was long.

Time to prioritize. What can I do first that will give me the biggest chunk of information the quickest? I had a child that looked pretty dead. If we brought him back from that, however, he would be the biggest save. My other patient was having an asthma attack, which could be difficult, but she held her own.

The pedi doc searched for a job to do. He sat in the spot I would be in for intubation. That would be most helpful.

I pointed to the blue bag on the floor with all my medical equipment stuffed inside.

"In the top of that bag is a compartment. Open the zipper and pull out the orange kit. That is all your intubation stuff."

269

I grabbed the heart monitor — again. I pulled the leads, stuck them on the kid's chest, and flipped the dial. Nothing. The light slid from left to right without a blip. This child had been in a fire for an extended period. This child was dead. The doctor, however, still wanted to try from the way he worked. Okay. We'll give it a shot.

My other patient sat on the bench, her hands on her knees, trying to sit straight and make her lungs as big as possible, working hard to breathe. I grabbed the oxygen bag, unzipped the outside pouch and pulled out the nebulizer. Most medicines were given through an IV. For asthmatics, I turned it into a mist. They just breathed it in.

I turned to grab the plastic vial of Albuterol out of the cabinet and checked in with the doctor.

"How're you doing?"

He glanced up at me, unsettled in the small space of the ambulance. In his left hand he gripped the laryngoscope blade, the tube in his right.

"I think I'm about ready."

I grabbed the vial, ripped off the top and turned back to my patient, speaking over my shoulder to the doctor, "I'll be with you by the time you get that tube."

I squirted the medicine into the chamber for misting, screwed on the top, hooked up the oxygen tubing and flipped the dial to eight liters. My patient took the nebulizer as the Albuterol misted out the end of the tube. She'd gone this route enough. She stuck the tube in her mouth and breathed the medicine as far into her lungs as possible. Held, released. Good.

I turned back to help the doctor.

Just in time. He drew the blade out of the child's mouth. The end of the plastic tube should be halfway to the kid's lungs. I leaned over the child and removed the pediatric bag-valve-mask from the cabinet, put it together and handed it to the doctor as he finished tying off the tube.

I hooked the stethoscope in my ears and listened while the doctor pressed a few rounds of air into the kid's lungs.

The air rushed clearly on both sides and nothing over the stomach. He was in the trachea putting air into the lungs, not the esophagus, and blowing up the stomach.

Chest compressions would be a good idea about now.

I took a position over the kid's chest and pressed down, then lifted, feeling his ribs spring back, down and up, starting a rapid pace to circulate oxygen the doctor now pushed into his lungs.

I could see with perfect clarity what we had here. I pounded on the body of a child from a smoked-up house fire with temperatures, at the floor, of several hundred degrees where he lay for at least twenty minutes. When I checked him the first time, on the sidewalk, he didn't have a pulse. By now we'd added five minutes, to be generous.

He was dead. Even the heart monitor said he was dead. But, I rationalized, this was a child. They pulled out of some horrible stuff. I pressed up and down on the kid's chest.

No. This isn't right. Anger boiled inside me. I had a very live patient sitting right next to me needing my attention. I was being distracted from helping someone. Yeah, he was a kid, but dead was dead. You didn't come back from dead.

Actually, in this business, there was almost dead, sorta dead and kinda dead. Those you can do something about. With this kid, being in the fire that long, he was dead dead and I just turned my back on my live patient to pound on a dead kid's chest.

Damn, I hated this job sometimes.

The doctor had him intubated. Now it was time to give some drugs. And not by starting an IV on this kid. That I was not going to do. We could give the medicines through the tube going into his lungs. While not as effective, we gave a bigger dose. It soaked in through the lung tissue. The doctor needed help. He didn't know where anything was and I couldn't reach the bag on the floor.

I pointed and said, "In the main section of the same blue bag is a bunch of drugs taped into a baggie. That is all the Code drugs."

The doc reached over and grabbed the bundle. He ripped into the bag and pulled out the epinephrine, fumbling with the box as he also tried to keep the kid ventilated. This wouldn't do.

I said, "Here. Let me open them. I'll feed them to you."

"Thanks," he said. With the kid tubed, the doc relaxed a little. This part seemed familiar to him, even in the back of an ambulance.

I stopped chest compressions long enough to pop open the box, assembled the syringe and handed it back to him. Technically, unless he took over responsibility for this patient, I was supposed to be pushing the meds. I'd worry about the finer points later. Now, I tried to balance too many things at once, emotionally and physically.

The doctor pushed the medicine down the tube, forcing it in using the breathing from the bag-valve-mask. I kept an eye on the heart monitor just in case any miracles came down the highway. Epinephrine, also known as adrenalin, made things faster, stronger, and bigger. We hoped to create a heartbeat out of the flat, green line on the screen.

I continued pressing on the boy's chest to circulate the epi for about a minute. I stopped compressions. Nothing.

I restarted compressions and checked the heart monitor again. The line bounced as it moved from left to right, but the timing synced perfectly with my compressions of his chest. Damn. I hoped for something. At least a bit.

I could see in his eyes he still wanted to believe.

"Let's try another epi," he said.

"Okay."

I ripped open another box and handed him the syringe. He pushed the medicine. We both scrutinized the monitor and this time we expected the same thing.

I stopped CPR to get a clean look at our patient's heart rhythm. The green dot flowed across the screen without interruption. He was dead. Nothing would change that. He had been in the fire too long.

I needed to finish, officially.

"Are we done here?"

The doctor took a second before nodding his head.

"Yeah. Yeah, we're done."

I don't know if he had ever pronounced a patient before. Maybe this was different doing it in the back of an ambulance only twenty-five yards from where the patient lived and played. This wasn't the hospital. Here we brought medicine to the patient, all of it.

"I'll take care of it from here. Thank you for your help."

I turned to face my other patient as the doctor crawled out of the ambulance.

The lady stared at the face of our boy, his eyes toward the ceiling, unblinking in the bright lights. She pulled the nebulizer away from her lips to speak,

"He is my nephew."

It hit me like a brick. The emotion stirred from my stomach, rose to my chest, through my neck, and to my eyes. I caught it quickly before it spilled out.

I was mad now. I was furious. I couldn't wrap my mind around it enough to know whom I was mad at, but the anger burned my face.

I brought two patients into my ambulance. My ambulance. This was where my patients received more than just medical care. My ambulance was a safe place where all the bad stuff went away, where I made things better.

In my ambulance I knew what was going to happen before it happened and I had the medicine, the training, and the know-how to fix it or run like hell to the hospital to hand it off to someone else. If something did pop up and surprise me, I knew my tools well enough to catch it before it fell. That was what I did. That was my job. My patients trusted me to make them better.

I screwed up. I brought a kid into my ambulance I had already checked out. I knew he was dead the first time I saw him. Nobody survived a fire like that. I put a dead kid into my ambulance. Dead people didn't go in my ambulance!

Sure, he was a kid. But, damn it, that is my job. It shouldn't make a difference. I had to have the guts to say, "Dead is dead." My emotions got in the way and I let the lady stare at her nephew while I pounded on his chest and a doctor stuffed a small garden hose into his mouth and down into his lungs.

Trying to resuscitate someone was not gentle. And this lady witnessed something no one should see done to a loved one, especially if it wouldn't work.

I searched for the right thing to say. Everything that came to mind sounded trite and didn't cover the enormity of what she witnessed at my hand.

"I'm sorry. He was in the fire too long."

The aunt had no tears. She drew the medicine into her lungs. When she exhaled, the mist rose lazily out the other end of the tube. I kept busy by checking her lung sounds. I put the stethoscope in my ears, held the bell at the back of her neck, softly prodded her to lean forward and slid it down her bare back.

I had a good stethoscope. It blocked out noise very well. Tonight it stopped more. With my eyes closed, I crawled inside that muted world to determine how the air moved in and out as the aunt breathed. I flowed through her lung passages and measured their diameter to see if the medicine had worked. I found quiet inside her lungs. I heard no wheezing and the air sounded clean and clear.

It was also safe. Nothing bad hid here. I was familiar with the tissues. I floated through the ever-decreasing size of the bronchioles with the capillaries at the end receiving clean oxygen and ridding carbon dioxide. It was a simple and good process. There was no death here. Not tonight. Not inside these lungs.

I couldn't stay. I couldn't hide. I took the scope out of my ears and opened my eyes. The lights glared brightly from the ceiling. The sound of working firefighters and their chain saws seeped through the walls of the ambulance.

I shifted to the eyes of the aunt and read sadness. She surveyed me. I hoped my eyes were open enough to show my aching. I wanted her to know, too.

"I'm sorry."

She nodded her head.

I must move on. I asked her, "How are you doing? How's your breathing?"

She pulled the nebulizer away. "It's better."

"Let me get you a crew to take you to the hospital? They can watch and make sure your lungs stay clear."

She said, "Yeah, I probably should. Can I go where they took the other kids?"

"Yes. They can take you there."

I brought my radio off my hip and keyed the mike. "Avery Command, Medic 17."

A voice came back through the microphone. "Medic 17. Go ahead."

"Avery Command, can you direct a Code 2 ambulance to my location? I'm at the intersection of Avery and Tuscany. This is for a shortness of breath."

The Incident Commander responded in a detached voice, "Copy, Medic 17. We'll send one your way."

I turned back to the aunt. "They're on their way. They shouldn't be too long. Do you feel like you could use another treatment?"

"Yes. I still feel a little short."

I took the nebulizer and filled the canister to start the mist flowing again. I then busied myself with the paperwork. I wanted to give the transporting crew a finished product.

Finally, the aunt was taken to the hospital. I stepped out of my ambulance, moved to a nearby parked car and, using the trunk as my desk, started the paperwork for the nephew.

Now that the aunt was gone, I stopped thinking of the boy as the nephew. He was a dead kid who died before I ever touched him. Now I had to describe the incident and

275

the efforts to try to revive him. I leaned against the car and began writing the chart.

"Patient presents brought out of house after being in smoke and fire environment for minimum of twenty minutes . . ."

When I finished his chart I picked up the chart of the girl who still lay under the bush.

"Patient presents brought out of house after being in smoke and fire environment for minimum of twenty minutes . . ."

I also made sure I still had the chart from the lady who tried to rescue the children.

But first I had to call my wife.

I dug out my cell phone and dialed the number. I lay over the car trunk, pretending to do the paperwork spread before me. Water from the hoses slid down the hill and eddied around my boots with the darkness still shattered by headlights, emergency lights, streetlights, and flashlights on the firefighters' coats. The fire had been extinguished. Light smoke and steam rose from the windows.

The phone rang and Camille answered. I spoke, my voice chipper, like any other night when I called home.

"Hi, honey, I . . . Oh, my God." The tears began.

CHAPTER 34

Thoughts In My Head

I've chosen mid-span for my New Year's celebration. The railing feels cold and damp with silent morning fog.

There is terrific contrast here: The infinite black, suffocating any conscious thought; set against pure, flawless white beyond the bridge railings.

The Bridge to the Golden Gate. Fitting, I suppose.

It's peaceful, the fog. It shuts out everything, solves everything, in an absolute swaddle which accepts entrance by a simple release.

The prospect of becoming white, to rid the black, is joyous.

I step over, holding until the right moment and the perfect Time has come...

Then I release.

Happy New Year.

CHAPTER 35

SOB (Shortness of Breath)

I knocked on the door and yelled, "Fire Department!"
No sounds came our way from inside.
"Is this the right address?" I asked Greg, my partner.
"Yep. 2051 Turk. We're in the right spot."
I banged on the door again.
"Ambulance!"
By now the fire engine crew stood behind me and it was time for a new plan. Forcible entry was next up on the dance card and I was about to make that very suggestion to the engine officer when a reminder phrase popped into my head, "Try before you pry."
I grasped the door knob. It turned easily in my hand and the door swung open.
I yelled, "Ambulance!" as I scanned the room. I didn't need anybody popping out from behind a door with a shotgun thinking intruders were coming to rob them.
I viewed the downstairs of the apartment and logged a single room; a doorway, probably leading to the kitchen; and the stairs headed to the upper floor.
Also evident was the hospital bed with the old lady sitting on its edge. She wore an oxygen mask but she still looked short of breath from our vantage point.
Greg and I snapped to action, crossed the room in two steps, and dropped our bags.
"Afternoon, ma'am. Are you having trouble breathing?"
The woman didn't say a word but shook her head while smiling.
I reached down for the pulse oximeter clip in the right pouch of the heart monitor while Greg opened his bag for access to our oxygen bottle. I needed to place the sensor on her finger faster than Greg could hook her up. I wanted a reading of her levels before adding supplemental oxygen.

I pressed open the clip, the red laser inside already glowing, and slipped the soft plastic over our patient's first finger. The laser's light would penetrate through and be picked up on the other side. The machine would read the color of the red blood cells and extrapolate the percentage of oxygen contained in those cells. It also gave me a constant reading of her pulse rate; a handy bonus instead of the expense and time of patching her up on the heart monitor.

Greg opened the oxygen bottle with the wrench from the green bag. He reached past the patient, unplugged the tubing from the machine on the floor and forced it on our tank. He spun the dial to fifteen liters per minute.

Just in time. My monitor glowed a solid reading of 93% and a pulse rate of 98. Those numbers weren't so bad. Anything below 95% should be augmented according to my protocols. She had been on eight liters with her oxygen; the extra from us should make the difference.

"Ma'am, is that better?"

She smiled at me.

Something wasn't right. Yes, she shook her head as I asked questions but I sensed I was missing something. Her eyes, bright and tracking my movements with purpose, told me she was alert.

"Ma'am, do you speak English?"

Again, she smiled and shook her head. The eyes didn't change. She hadn't understood a word since we walked in the door.

Oh, well, I'd had language barriers with my patients before. The plan remained unchanged: Load her up in the chair and out to the ambulance. Also, by then we might be able to find her ID, medications, and a relative to fill us in a little more on what they had seen change to call 911.

I didn't know where the fire engine guys had gone. I think they were upstairs. Maybe they'd found a family member.

Greg positioned the stair chair next to our lady. We assisted her over, then snapped the belts around her chest and lap. I smiled at her a lot, spoke to her like she could understand me, and mostly just put her hands across her legs and patted them conveying the message I wanted her to keep them there when we carried her down the stairs.

I pushed the chair across the carpet and out the front door with Greg's help until a shrill voice behind me caused me to stop.

"What are you doing?!"

I guessed it was a relative.

"We're loading her into the ambulance. I'm glad we found you, I've got a few questions about what you saw and what has changed for you to call us."

"Bring her back inside!"

"Excuse me?"

"Bring her back inside and put her back in bed. She's not who I called you about. My son is upstairs. He's the one having trouble breathing."

"Oh."

Well, this was a new one.

Once I fully grasped the situation I still had questions.

"This woman doesn't look like she's doing too well, either."

"She's fine. She's always like that."

"Are you sure?"

"Yes. Put her back in bed."

"Okay, then."

And we wheeled her back inside.

"Greg, can you put her back in bed? I should go upstairs and find out what's wrong with our real patient."

"Sure."

Barely able to conceal his laughter, Greg stayed behind with our elderly "almost" patient while I grabbed the medical bag and took the stairs two at a time.

Upstairs I found a young man, about twenty-five, whose distinctive facial features suggested developmental disabilities. Watching his neck muscles strain and the skin draw in with each breath told me I had also located my patient. I grabbed my stethoscope out of the bag and took a listen to his lungs down the back of his shirt. I heard slight wheezing but with plenty of air surrounding those sounds. Easy fix. A little Albuterol and this boy would be fixed up in short order.

I directed the firefighters to assemble a breathing treatment for our guy. They had done this countless times over the years so I turned to the lady who stopped me from kidnapping the downstairs resident.

"Hi. Sorry about that. It's quite usual for us to go to the first patient who looks like they need us. So, this gentleman, what's the story?"

"His name is John. He's my son and he has asthma. He ran out of his inhalers the other day and we haven't been able to fill them yet. He's been getting more short of breath all day now."

I smiled a soft smile, trying to make up for my mix-up and signaling confidence we could take care of her son.

"We're giving him a breathing treatment and that should clear him up. I still think he should go to the hospital to make sure everything stays in order and they can also refill his prescription while you're there. Do you have his ID? Where are his medicines and what hospital do you want him to go to?"

"Yes, here's his ID." She handed me his medical cards. "His inhaler is on the table. That's all he uses. And, please, can we go to Cal-Pac?"

"Is John his own conservator? Does he sign for himself?"

Anybody who had legal rights issues as a part of their life knew what I was talking about.

"No. I'm his conservator. I'll be going to the hospital."

"Which brings me to the woman downstairs . . ."

"Yes, she's my mother."

"Your mother! Well, you've got quite a lot going on here, don't you?" I made sure I gave her my most caring smile to let her see my sincerity about her home's workload. This woman deserved sainthood. She had a full plate and yet she took it in good stride. I was impressed.

"It is a lot, but I do what I can."

"And you are doing it well. Can your mother stay here by herself? We can bring her along if we need to."

"No, she's fine to be alone for a bit."

"Okay, then. Shall we get going to the hospital . . . with the correct patient?"

"Yes, thank you."

And we got the patient into the ambulance for a short ride to the hospital.

Note to self: Make sure to do a full scene size-up before committing to a plan.

CHAPTER 36

Christmas With The Eberharts

Another year has passed. Like dodging hurricanes in a tumultuous sea, the Good Ship Eberhart, once again readies for the holiday season. The kids are bailing water, the dog is up to his nose and paddling, but Camille and Scott still smile and put on suntan lotion from the poop deck.

In fine tradition let's begin with Scott. The San Francisco Fire Department hasn't uncovered any solid evidence why he should be fired. They obviously have not looked under the rug.

Scott moved to more upscale pastures in the Pacific Heights district of the City. Yes, this is the neighborhood of the same name as an unsettling movie starring Michael Keaton, who plays the renting thorn in a building owner's side. This is also the neighborhood of Robin Williams' movie "Mrs. Doubtfire." The point is, this ain't the Projects anymore and there are just not enough people getting shot and stabbed nearby. Although drunk rich people can be fun.

The Department finally recognized that Scott is both a firefighter and a paramedic. He is performing both duties and they often send him "down the hill" to the Marina District, to ride the fire engine at another hardship station. On the upside, Scott is becoming quite celebrated for his excellent desserts. He loves to make pies and cookies.

Camille is done with school. They didn't even have to kick her out. She finished on her own. This may come as a surprise, but Camille did not slow down. She still does medical record review for a law firm in San Francisco. It's a pretty sweet deal. They FedEx her records, she reviews them, collates the data into a readable format, and emails the product back to the firm. They FedEx more records and she bills them a lot of money, if she so chooses, all while wearing a bathrobe. On occasion Camille also still performs as an expert witness. She hasn't actually made it to court. If she does, she may faint. To justify her expert status, Camille still works a few days a month at Santa Rosa Memorial Hospital.

Beyond all this legal stuff, Camille still manages to find time to volunteer in the kids' classrooms, go to the gym, manage the kids when Scott is at work (or even when Scott is not at work), cook every once in a while, and keep us all in line. Scott continues to watch her spin, catch the parts that fall off, and putter in his own projects like riding his bicycle 450 miles from Montreal to Boston again and painting an undersea mural in the kids' bathroom. That project is rumored to be finished sometime within the year.

Justine, sixteen years old, has blossomed. The parental units no longer have a child. They gained a functioning, conversational, and pleasant housing partner. She scored something akin to an apartment due to last year's house remodel and now, although it may not be wise, Justine's bedroom is next to the garage. She decides when she will deign to eat with the Commoners, uses her own bathroom, and only comes upstairs when she wants something; invariably while her mother is trying frantically to complete her committed hours. Thank God Justine is pleasant, responsible, and without any documented vices. All this freedom could be ugly with some other child.

Justine also went on a date where the boy came by the house to pick her up. Scott was at work and missed the first opportunity for young man hazing. She continued to make friends by challenging another young man to a taco eating contest — and winning. The final fun thus far is Justine is now in possession of a license issued by the State of California.

Oh, God.

Elise, eight years old, and Kylene, six and a half, are doing great. They are in third and second grade, respectively. Their intended teachers retired or got promoted, which gives them both new teachers. Luckily, both seem to be good with children. Beyond school, the kids are staying active as usual.

We pried them away from gymnastics as it was getting too expensive and no one seemed destined to challenge for the Olympics. We replaced this with soccer. They were on different teams, which added to the scheduling joy.

Kylene's team, co-coached by Dad, did a lot of learning and had fun. Translated as, they didn't win a game but enjoyed playing. At this age, they don't keep score yet.

Elise's team, the one not co-coached by Dad, came in second for her league. Elise loves it and their whole team signed up together to play indoor soccer through January. Scott was volunteered to be relief coach in case a scheduling snafu or a biblical plague came to pass and wiped out the other two coaches.

Both girls are also still going strong on the piano front. Kylene is following right on the heels of Elise by moving into practice books as Elise finishes them. Elise graduated from the venerable Lady Up The Street and is now with The Lady Across Town. Elise made the shift well and is still enjoying it. Scott and Camille will drop money for that.

Elise is destined for braces. It helps that another friend is going through the same. She is slated for a year of adjustment. Camille and Scott get to pay for it. Justine is out of her braces. Kylene will probably join the team soon.

Kylene began the year keeping us entertained. She was counting palm trees. Yes, just that. They would be the same palm trees every day. She would count them every time they were passed while en route to wherever. Northern California does not have a lot of palm trees. It's not what this part of the state is famous for. No matter. Kylene was intent on counting all of them. She did quit after a few months. She got tired when she reached a respectable number, somewhere around twelve thousand, two thousand, four hundred and seventy-two. Note the number. Yes, it is written correctly as Kylene counted it.

To round out the organic members of the family, Keyan is still ready and willing to make puppies. He hasn't gotten the phone call lately. Canine Companions, a local agency for assistance dogs, tell us they are evaluating the quality of his offspring in regards to percentage graduating. He hits their mark and he gets more phone calls for service (so to speak). He isn't producing enough successful graduates? Things are cut off. If he only realized, he should be filled with performance anxiety. Instead, Keyan remains consistent with his "Does anybody want to play with me?" look.

The cats are the hit of the year. Thomas is reaching new widths. He is nineteen pounds and lies on his side rather than on his stomach. His breathing would be impeded if he did otherwise. He is fat and happy, as the saying goes. Mostly, he is happy because Blackie has been evicted. Blackie chose to do unsightly things — a lot — in a corner of the living room. Camille was not overjoyed and now the Black One resides in the garage next to the food. Blackie, ever the king, refuses to acknowledge this as a step down. Thomas does the snooty thing as he eats his fill and then waddles past Blackie to be let inside. Oh, the psychological issues and hierarchies of cats.

As mentioned, Justine is now in possession of a valid State of California driver's license. She did not achieve her freedom of driving without her own moments that need to be recounted for all to hear and for posterity. On to this year's story.

There was not much question who would assist in her driver's education. Her mother is a wee bit tense with those inevitable close calls that are standard with a teen driver. That left Scott.

Scott teaches evasive driving. Scott is used to nearly being killed by excitable partners trying on the new suit of high-performance driving. So Scott is on the freeway with Justine, telling her, "Come on, put your foot in it, you're not even doing the speed limit yet."

Scott and Justine began in a church parking lot. It was decided for her that Justine should learn to drive a stick. The first time Justine got going from a standstill Scott let her motor around a little and then asked her to stop. She did. Rather quickly.

Scott said, after he got over the whiplash, "When you stop you need to push the clutch in so the car won't stall."

Justine's response?

"Every time? That's silly. Why?"

That was a tough one in the heat of the moment.

"I don't know. You just do."

Justine became at ease when Scott would laugh as she stalled the car, then attempted to wear the gear box down into little metal shavings. Soon, Justine was doing third gear in the parking lot with Scott reminding her to give the wall a little more room as she rounded the corner.

Next, Justine progressed to a local neighborhood. Only one time did she blow the stop sign while making a right hand turn and we had to avoid the other car. She was doing very well. From then it was off to anywhere we could find.

Justine and Scott had many wonderful trips around the county. Justine would say, "Where to?" Scott would say, "I don't care." Justine would say, "Where does that road go?" Scott would say, "Let's find out." Many of these drives were in the evening and after dark. Thus it was for one.

Justine and Scott were making a trip out Sonoma Highway. This is a gorgeous, bucolic road with "scenic drive" designation. The soft, winding turns showcase some lovely vineyards, mountains, and trees one can't see at night. To prevent the need for camping gear, Scott did maintain a sense of location and made some suggestions that would generally keep us making a circle that would end up at home eventually. It was one of those turns Scott was looking for.

Madrone Road is well marked—for a country road. Scott knew it was coming up soon. Scott mentioned we would be taking a right turn. In the dark, Scott became disoriented at the wrong moment as a road came up swiftly out of the darkness. Scott made a quick calculation and decided we weren't too late.

"Justine, turn here. Turn right."

And she did. Quite well. Justine executed a rapid deceleration combined with a sharp right hand turn, bringing the car to the new road in swift fashion. However.

Yeah, however.

As Justine was doing this maneuver in a short moment of space and time, she knocked the light switch, thus turning off the headlights. The mind is an incredible thing. In the short second before everything went totally black, Scott noted they were not on Madrone Road. They were in the driveway of Bruce Cohn's winery, the manager for the Doobie Brothers, by the way. Before blackness consumed all outside view, Scott saw that Mr. Cohn had decided to split his driveway. Thus, the road ended, the grass began, then stopped shortly at the roots of a large oak tree.

"Stop! Justine, stop! Tree! Tree!"

And she did.

It was at that moment Scott knew Justine was going to do just fine as a driver and she just had to jump through a few hoops required by the State.

Happy Holidays to all. Until next year.

The Eberharts

CHAPTER 37

The Removal

There it was on the dispatch computer screen. In print.
Respond for the Cock Ring Removal.

This would be interesting.

The patient met us at the door, late twenties, bald, clean shaven, and quite probably naked under the towel wrapped around his waist post-shower style. The fire engine crew consisted of Tony and me along with two women, Kerry and Maribeth, whom the patient vetoed from making entrance. The fact he could a) summon the strength to meet us at the door and b) become selective about certain aspects of his rescuers, told me volumes that his issue did not immediately threaten his life – or limb, so to speak. If I needed the ladies' help, I could overrule him later. The ambulance, with Josh and Michael, arrived soon after and we all convened, minus the ladies, upstairs in the living room.

The patient opened our meeting by suggesting the first item to be addressed.

"Dude! Get this thing off me!"

I liked to use a phrase in situations like this, one that kept things in perspective and helped me stay relaxed and able to do my job—problem solving—with the utmost efficiency: "This is not my emergency."

Because of that mantra, my response was purposefully calm and quietly directive.

"Sir, sit down and let's see what we've got here."

"Where! Where should I sit?!"

"There," pointing to the closest dining room chair, "will do fine."

The man sat and unfolded his towel.

As noted at the front door, our patient had chosen to be bald. He had also chosen, now easily apparent, to carry this grooming technique to all aspects of his personage.

Excellent.

The problem was obvious.

The purpose of a cock ring is to impede the movement of blood, after circulating into the penis and causing erection, preventing it from flowing back out. This impedance causes further engorgement, enlarging the penis, an aspect with which many men seem to be obsessed. The constriction of the penis also slows and heightens the orgasmic action and sensation. Every man is definitely on board for that.

Our man had donned his cock ring completely against his torso, as recommended. The wearer, or his partner, achieves this by gently grasping the scrotum and slipping one testicle at a time through the ring. Then, due to the incredibly acrobatic folding abilities of a flaccid penis, the head is driven through the same hole.

Over time, and beyond the suggested donning period, the stainless-steel ring had done its job of reducing blood flow, causing our patient's penis and scrotum to attain a darkish blue color. More problematic was his scrotum, which had swollen to about the size of a softball. The ring, about the diameter able to accommodate a golf ball, was obviously not coming off with any amount of coaxing the way it had gone on. To fully investigate the possibilities, the EMT from the ambulance slipped a finger, gloved, between the ring and the scrotum. The patient howled at that slightest of touch.

"How long has this thing been on?" I asked.

"About two hours! Am I damaged?"

"Nah, in the case of cuts and other reduced blood flow situations, you've got about six hours before it truly becomes a problem. You're good."

The man's eyes got bigger.

"Well, maybe longer. More like four to five hours. I put it on, then I fell asleep. Get this thing off!"

Hmmm. Yes, closer to 'crunch time.' But the color didn't appear that bad yet. He still had some blood flow, not total occlusion.

"You're still good, man. Let's see what we can do."

"I've been trying myself. I tried pliers and a hammer."

That made me wince.

We still had options to weigh and a plan to devise. The four of us rescuers stepped a few feet away and I started.

"So, any ideas?"

I looked to Michael, the EMT, and Josh, the medic, and spelled out the most obvious of plans.

"You two could transport him to the hospital. They're going to call the Rescue Squad when you arrive, from the same Department who employs me, and those guys carry pretty much the same tools we do. At least those with which you would want to approach this problem. I'd say that leaves out the cutting torch."

"How about a ring cutter?" said Tony, standing by me.

"Excellent idea."

I rummaged around in our bag and pulled out the ring cutter. Ring removal from fingers is common enough that we carry a little hand-held, manually operated circular saw. One look at the small teeth of the cutter and the stainless steel of the ring caused me to drop it back in the bag. Next.

Michael piped in.

"I live right across the street."

"Really? What have you got?" I asked.

"A Dremel tool."

I did too and used it often on my dog's toenails. Using the hand-held miniature circular saw and whirring right through the metal ring sounded simple and quick.

"Nice. Go get it."

The rest of us kept the patient company and struck up a conversation.

"You know," said Josh, "they make these out of rubber."

I stifled a smirk.

I needed to step outside and make sure I was thinking of all angles. At the top of the stairs lay a pair of pliers and a hammer. I created a mental picture of our man sitting on the landing, his "package" in free swing as he desperately worked at the issue, trying to find leverage, attempting different positions for a backstop to his efforts and fighting the nausea from the pain.

I winced and walked down the stairs.

Outside, I met Kerry and Maribeth chatting away the time and Maribeth made the effort to point out, with a smile, they were being discriminated against.

"Yes, you are," was my response.

"So, how's it going in there?"

I formed an "O" with my hands to softball size.

"His scrotum."

The women cringed.

At that moment Michael came back across the street empty-handed.

"Where's the Dremel?"

"I couldn't find it."

"Hmmm. Let's see. What else do we have?"

As I mentally ran over our list of tools on the fire engine, Tony came downstairs and I told him we needed another idea. He thought for a brief second before coming up with the answer. I grinned at the suggestion, opened up the cabinet, and removed them from their perch. Bolt cutters.

Thinking out loud, I voiced my next concern.

"We need a barrier of some sort."

Kerry spoke up.

"I keep a piece of plastic behind the driver's seat."

"Yeah, that'll work."

"I won't want it back when you're done."

I found the plastic while Tony threw the bolt cutters over his shoulder, then he and Michael headed upstairs. Out of courtesy for Kerry and her plastic, as I stepped back inside, I cut off a size I thought we would need. Of course I pocketed the rest without telling Kerry. I couldn't just hand it back to her without her thinking I had used it. This call swelled with joke material.

All male personnel reconvened by the patient. Josh and Michael liked Tony's idea and tool selection, but we decided a horizontal surface would be better for this procedure, so we all relocated to the bedroom.

Let's take a moment to wholly understand the problem and the thoughts for execution of the solution. Again, this man's scrotum was engorged to about the size of a softball. His penis, now decidedly flaccid, was not an issue and only had to be held out of the way for better viewing. The perineum, the area below the scrotum, had become very tender to touch or manipulation.

Our selected tool was a set of small 24-inch heavy-duty bolt cutters constructed of drop-forged steel, weighing in at 5.6 pounds (2.6 kilograms), and possessing a 7/16-inch cutting range for soft materials but reducing to a 3/8-inch range for medium hard issues. Our cock ring, constructed of stainless steel approximately 3/16 of an inch in thickness, resided well within the specs for our tool to handle.

"Dude! Hurry up! Get this thing off me!"

"Relax. We're working on it. We're going to use bolt cutters." And Tony displayed our removal device. "Lie back on the bed."

"You're going to use those?"

"Sure. We very carefully slide them on the ring, make a snip, place them again on the other side of the ring, another snip and we're done."

"I don't care, man. Just get this off."

Our patient sat back, feet on the floor, and propped himself up by his elbows.

Nope. I couldn't get a clear shot at his genitals and I said, more to the other workers in the room, "This isn't going to work." Then, louder, to the patient, "Scoot back. Bend your knees and put your feet on the edge of the bed."

There. The penis, scrotum, and cock ring were much more accessible. Excellent.

"Hurry!! I can't take this." And our guy started rocking back and forth in his agony. "God damn it! Get this thing off me! The pain, I'm going to be ruined!"

"Hey. You're going to have to hold still while we do this."

"This thing is killing me!" More writhing.

I stepped back and looked at Josh.

"This isn't going to work. We need to calm this guy down. Any ideas? I mean, we could give him Valium."

Josh said, "Nah, let's work with him a bit."

Yeah, he was right. Let's not be so free with the drugs.

"Dude, slow down. We're working with bolt cutters, here. We don't want to slip and cut the wrong stuff."

"Just get this fucker off me!"

Okay, then. Tony was our bolt cutter guy. I took the plastic, a piece from an old jug of vegetable oil and slipped the small sliver between the ring and his scrotum. I had to wiggle it a bit.

"Aaaagh! Shit! Hurry, damn it! That hurts!"

It was quite amazing how everything became professional. I was staring, from about one foot away, at my efforts to place a plastic shim between some guy's balls and his taint. Michael held the penis out of the way and Tony was ready to perform delicate surgery with a pair of two-foot-long bolt cutters.

"Aaaaagh!" Our patient expressed.

"Okay, Tony, I think we're ready down here."

A consummate professional, Tony delicately introduced the bolt cutters to the cock ring. He spread the mouth wide and got a firm purchase. I examined his placement. He'd gotten a healthy chunk of cock ring firmly in the cutters with the plastic shim held in place and no flesh anywhere near. Well, relatively, it was all close quarters. Tony was ready to close the handles on my signal.

"Hold still."

I pointed at Tony.

With a firm squeeze, the handles came together, the mouth closed and the cut was made.

Later, Kerry told me the scream could be heard outside.

"Aaaaaaaaaaaaaaaagh!!!

The cut was successful and no essential items were damaged.

"Get it off, get it off, get it off!" And he tried to sit up.

I pushed him back to the bed. He didn't get it. The job was only half done.

"We have to make another cut."

"What?! Can't you pry it off?"

"No. We can't bend it. Besides, that would hurt like a mother . . . . "

"It's already killing me."

"Lie back. We'll make another cut and the whole thing will fall away."

Reluctantly, he lay back on the bed.

"Just hurry. I can't take this much longer."

I moved the shim to the other side of the ring. This time Michael used a little lube. Hey, that got the shim in easier. The things we learned along the way.

"Okay, Tony."

The cutters were placed once again, the shim ensured to be doing its job, all flesh confirmed at a safe distance.

"Go."

Tony performed his practiced technique and I noted it did take a bit of squeezing while also not rocking the cutters too much. Well done, Tony.

Splang!

The cock ring separated and the two pieces flew across the room. Wow, wasn't expecting that. Glad no one got hit. That would have been hard to explain.

The job was done. The man's genitalia were now his own, once again.

"Okay, sir." On to the next step in this process. "Which hospital do you want to go to?"

"I don't want to go to the hospital."

I was a little taken aback and I shifted into legal mode.

"Well, sir. I have no idea what kind of damage you might have caused here. I mean, yes, everything is looking back towards normal, but you had reduced blood flow to . . . well, a rather sensitive area for quite a long time."

"Yeah, but it's looking normal now, right? I can use it, right?"

"Yeah, but, seriously, do you want to mess around with this? I have no idea what risks you are taking."

"Nope. I'm not going."

Josh stepped in and turned to me. "I'll take it from here. If we can convince him to go, we're on our way. If not, I'll involve everybody from the Pope on down to cover our asses. You guys can go."

"Alright."

I turned to the patient. "Good luck with that." Pointing at his crotch.

Tony hefted the bolt cutters over his shoulder and we headed downstairs, past the hammer and pliers.

CHAPTER 38

Two Worlds Entwined

One shift I took half the day off to play some saxophone. The band started in the morning, playing in a restaurant along the piers of San Francisco. In the afternoon we set up and rocked out for a birthday party down on the peninsula. The sax sounded awesome and the music rose from within as I hit a few good licks. God, I love that feeling.

When I got to the station, the tones went off almost as soon as I walked in the door. It was for an assault. Some lady got beat up by her husband. I trusted the guy working for me checked out the rig and I jumped in while James buckled in on the driver's side. I heard the back door swing open and shut as a young man sat in the jump seat in the back.

"Who's he?" I asked James.

"He's a ride along we've had all day."

"EMT? Medic student?"

"Nah, just someone wondering what the job is all about."

"Okay."

I yelled to the back as James turned on the siren, "Welcome, my name is Scott."

"Hi, Scott. I'm Robert. Anything you want me to do? Anything you want me to grab?"

"You just follow James and me. Grab what we tell you to grab and stay right next to me. If we start to run away, make sure you're in the ambulance first."

I threw a quick smile at him and turned forward to make sure we got to the scene safely. Out of the corner of my eye I saw Robert crane his neck to see out the front windshield.

James drove, one hand on the steering wheel, weaving between cars, finishing the sandwich he'd apparently been trying to eat for two hours. Tossing down the last bite, he cleanly avoided a large truck. I sat in the passenger seat, calling out "Clear right!" ensuring our safe travel through the red lights, at least from my side of the ambulance.

We pulled up to the address. I got out and grabbed the jump kit, still fighting a surreal realization that a few hours ago I was grooving and dancing with a group of partiers and now I was stepping into a home where screaming and fists were probably a nightly occurrence. Outside the one-room apartment, a man sat cuffed on the porch being questioned by a cop. I continued past because I wasn't here for him.

Inside, more cops pointed me to the woman on the couch. I counted out her pulse and took a blood pressure before I cleaned her head wound, catalogued the bruises and swelling on her face, and told her,

"Leave the guy. You're worth more than this. It's going to get worse. He may even kill you."

I then turned and soothed the anxieties of the frightened children who stood no more than the height of the gun holsters worn about the room.

Back at the station after the call, I checked out the ambulance. Robert asked questions and wondered what everything did. I opened the cabinets as I did inventory and showed him how each was split into categories such as airway and bandaging. I taught him how to take a blood pressure and how the heart monitor worked. I even patched him up to show his own rhythm and ran a strip, a souvenir of sorts.

His eyes glowed with the fire I once had. He had the yearning to know everything and witness something fantastic. I still had passion inside me. It had softened and I could now walk onto a scene and categorize the chaos and decipher the drama flying around the room to create a list of what needed to be done.

As for the callous feelings creeping up? After thirty years of doing this job, I should expect to be a little desensitized to bodies by now. They were dead. I could write a chart about the last minutes of their life.

Sometimes I silently hoped they stayed dead despite our efforts. Was I playing God? No. I have destroyed ninety-year-old ladies with chest compressions. I have given drugs to raise a heartbeat in someone who has been living in a vegetative state from a stroke for months. A failure in our attempts to resuscitate that person is not losing the fight. On those people, a returning pulse is knowing I stopped a door from closing that should be allowed to shut and will anyway in a few weeks after much pain and hundreds of thousands of dollars.

It was the living I still had to be aware of. I still believed in humanity. I knew what I could offer and maybe I was quicker to know when the patient's needs were beyond my toolbox. That was still a person on my gurney. I still had something to contribute.

A long time ago I treated a guy shot seven times who died on the way to the hospital. His soul, his essence of humanity, slipped out of the ambulance, like a trapeze artist failing his partner's grip, to leave me delivering a fleshy corpse to the ED staff. I had been his last chance to remain whole and I was sure I failed him. I wondered if I wanted to wade into that kind of anguish anymore.

Luckily, that doesn't happen every day. In between the crazy calls I've solved a few problems, offered a hand up when that was all that was needed, laughed a little at the things people did, and threw out a smile on a rainy day. When something big did come in I was part of a team doing amazing things. The bad calls weren't going to stop and if weird things were going to happen, I wanted to be the guy they called to solve it. I still wanted to offer the grasp from the trapeze and lift my patient to the safety of the platform high above the circus floor. I still wanted to play the game.

Every once in a while a hard call happened and we all gathered around the table to talk about it and debrief. I believed in that process. I likened stress to the roots of a weed. Letting them grow made them difficult to remove. Dig them out fast, as soon as the seeds are sown. Talk about the call. Talk about it a lot. Eventually, the telling became just another story.

Robert watched as I put the monitor leads away and then he asked,

"Earlier today everyone wore their uniform shirts and now they're in t-shirts while you're still wearing the one with the badge on it. Why?"

"I like to wear my uniform shirt until I go to bed because I'm the paramedic. When I walk in the door I'm selling a product: My knowledge and my ability to rein in whatever is wrong. I want people to meet someone dressed nicely. I want them to know when we come through the door; things are going to get better. I want them to let go of their problem."

"Yeah, that makes sense. I also noticed you and James are the only two with patches on your sleeves."

"In the San Francisco Fire Department the firefighters don't have patches. The Department never designed one. When we merged into the fire department, they made one for the paramedics.

"A long time ago, a partner once told me I would own a Yamaha. He stole the phrase from an old motorcycle commercial and meant I would own a paramedic patch and be proud to wear it.

"I have earned this patch. I have done a few things and seen a few things over the years to keep it. I'd say, yeah, I own a Yamaha."

Afterword

These are the stories of my career . . . so far. As I finish this book, I have been inside the Emergency Medical Services industry for over thirty years, twelve in the privates and twenty-six in the fire department. Today my plans are to shoot for a total of forty-two years with sirens in my ears.

I still love going to work. On some level I don't know why I'm the lucky one still alive in the business. There are ups and downs, ins and outs. There are patients whom I wanted to leave in their own self-destructive anger. Others I will never forget because their grasp on their condition and humanity touched me in a way that was perfect on that day.

Am I sane? Have I been irreparably altered? I think the answer to both is "Yes." To cope with what I am expected to see, some of me has been dulled. At the same time, those experiences made me find life precious, notice miracles every day, and believe in the importance to put out the effort of just a little kindness that can make a huge difference to someone on the right day.

I have lived through dark passages. To avoid those places in the future, I analyzed the pieces creating the mosaic of those moments. A common denominator did show up. Sleep deprivation puts me in a place I don't like to be. I bottom out at a certain level and can function but I interact with others in survival mode. My kids tell a story of how I forgot to pick them up from school one day. I didn't forget. I sat down on the couch and woke up when the school called.

I'm also a firm believer in incident stress debriefing. People and scenes float in my head and will never leave. Even telling those stories today evokes a tightening of the throat and a welling of tears. But those events don't control my life. Those with me at the debriefing sessions saved me from that. I'm sure the psychology of stress management will change and evolve. For what we know today, this seems to work for me.

There is someone to whom I am deeply indebted. Every married person thanks their spouse for the support and love needed to write a book. I am equally thankful for that, and not only that. My wife has kept me sane in this crazy business. She is my true debriefing crew. The phone call to her after I had pronounced four children dead was the factor allowing me to go into the official debriefing and support others instead of me needing to be patched together.

She is a nurse, and a damn good one. She worked in the emergency room for a large portion of my time on the ambulance. She knows what I do, the stresses I witness. She declares she could never do my job. Likewise, I could never do her job.

In all the other aspects of our lives, she is amazing. We've had many fun discussions about the ability of the female of our species to multitask and the inability of the male of our species to do so. I'm sure some men out there are whizzes. I am not one of them. Watching her manage the kids, the house, and her sixteen jobs at one time and still be a wonderful person is breathtaking.

The Christmas letters are written to family and friends and I changed the content very little. The young folks who taught me the skill of fatherhood are three amazing people and I am always proud of them. They are now young adults and they are one of the reasons I wrote this book. I wanted to explain why I was late picking them up from school that day. I also wanted to explain why some days I was sad at dinner and needed an extra hug.

The chapter, "I'm Not In Charge" told the story of a young girl. As an adult, she gave me permission to present her story. I changed the addresses and scenarios of most. I changed the names of all. On a few, the nosebleed lady for one, some of her mannerisms were a compilation of many patients whose couches I've sat on while we sifted through the details for far longer than seemed necessary, or possible. I'm happy some of those people live inside of me. Others provide cautionary tales or memories of survival.

An interesting note on the chapter "Thoughts In My Head." I was a member of a fantastic writing website, "Thenextbigwriter.com." That chapter was a writing challenge to create a story with exactly 100 words. I'll wait while you go back and count the words.

The reason for writing this book is multi-pronged. For the emergency medical professional, it can be a source of laughter and commiseration at having dealt with the "same stuff, different day." For the newbies to the EMS world, it can serve as a text for what they are about to get into. For my family, I wanted a memory of my career. For the general public, I wanted to show what really happens inside an ambulance.

The paramedics and EMTs who live among you will corroborate what I talk about. When they do, watch their eyes. They'll drift off to another place, another street corner, another car, another room, to remember someone rattling around in their head. They might not want to tell you about it; to save you from the graphics, to save themselves from some pain, or to save you from a sick sense of black humor. But the love and patience they have for their job, humanity in general, and the people they are tasked to care for at any moment on any shift is real. Give them a hug. Not because they're "heroes." I'm not a hero. They deserve a hug because tomorrow, when they wake up, they're going to put on their uniform and do it again.

Thank you to all who provided material for this project, either as a patient, a partner, or family. It's been a long, strange trip, and I'm not done yet.

About the Author

As a well-rounded individual, Scott Eberhart is a lot of things. He is a husband to an amazing woman who runs circles around him in almost everything. He is a father to three young adults who all have apparently joined society as productive members. In other words, a parent's dream.

He plays saxophone, has stumbled up to owning four, or five, if you count the one residing with one of the kids, and still fumbles around on flute. He plays music well enough to be in bands and play weddings, bar and bat mitzvahs, and funerals. Fun Fact: Whenever you see a rock band and there is a flute on stage, to be played will either be a Jethro Tull simulation or Van Morrison's "Moondance."

His retirement dream is to sit in the corner of a cafe with a saxophone and get ignored.

But, most of this book has delved into Scott's life in Emergency Medical Services.

Scott is aiming for forty-two years with sirens. He no longer works on ambulances or even fire engines. He is still with the San Francisco Fire Department as a Paramedic Captain in the EMS6 Division. He spends his afternoons and nights, mostly in the Tenderloin, looking for clients who call 911 the most. He is charged with getting to know them… very well. He attempts to improve their lives using tricks, cajoling, sheer stubbornness, parenting techniques, and the occasional purchase of a slice of pizza. The resulting goal is the clients get improved lives and the system loses a 911 client. Our #1 client has an "emergency" eighteen times a month. It's fascinating work and should keep Scott satisfied another few years.

Besides, Scott is under the direction he is not allowed to retire until he has a hobby and three friends already retired.

Music appears to be the hobby.